THROUG...

Teachings of the 20 Mysteries of the Rosary and the Herbs and Foods Associated with Them

BY GAIL FAITH EDWARDS

The information shared in this book is intended for educational purposes. The author and publisher are not responsible for any adverse effects or consequences resulting from the use of any remedies, procedures or preparations included in *Through the Wild Heart of Mary; Teachings of the 20 Mysteries of the Rosary and the Herbs and Foods Associated with Them*

Photos: Laura Grace Hilmer, pgs. 11, 290
Rosa Jane Fangboner, pgs. 39, 43, 46, 53, 206, 285, 297, 353
Gail Faith Edwards, pgs. 15, 17, 35, 45, 58, 59, 72, 77, 83, 205, 225, 229, 231, 252, 273, 275, 280, 292, 301, 321, 351
Jess Clancy pgs. 354, 357

Watercolors: Gail Faith Edwards, pgs. 3, 6, 9, 12, 14, 16, 19, 23, 32, 41, 42, 51, 61, 69, 78, 91, 93, 103, 105, 107, 111, 112, 121, 135, 137, 147, 149, 153, 164, 165, 166, 167, 168, 169, 170, 171, 172, 173, 174, 176, 177, 178, 179, 180, 182, 183, 184, 185, 186, 187, 189, 192, 193, 194, 195, 196, 197, 198, 199, 200, 202, 203, 215, 216, 222, 228, 232, 235, 240, 244, 245, 246, 265, 274, 277, 284, 294, 295, 296, 299, 316, 317, 319, 324, 331, 349, 350, 358, 359, 364, 366

Scans: Gail Faith Edwards, pgs. 340, 342, 351

Line drawings: Lynne Harwood, pgs. 210, 264, 305

Illustrations: pgs. 29, 30, 33, 38, 49, 56, 65, 114, 217, 237, 250, 251, 269, 270, 278 - Every attempt has been made to credit the original source. If we have inadvertently used an image of yours please notify the publisher and full credit will be given in the next edition.

Cover art, book design and layout: Gail Faith Edwards
Book cover design, BookCover Pro

Preface ©2009 by Michael J. Caduto. All Rights Reserved.

No part of this book may be reproduced without the author's permission except small excerpts to be used for promotional material only.

Library of Congress Control Number: 2009903549

ISBN 978-09753022-7-9

The author welcomes your correspondence - gailea88@gmail.com

www.blessedmaineherbs.com
www.studyherbalmedicines.com

Bertha Canterbury/Rosina Publishing
Athens, Maine 04912

Copyright 2009 Gail Faith Edwards

This book is dedicated
to my children

Rosa,
whose love and care are boundless.

Grace,
the essence of devotion.

Belle,
who shares her joy of living.

And Johnny, Kasia and Alex,
who bravely led us all into the next generation.

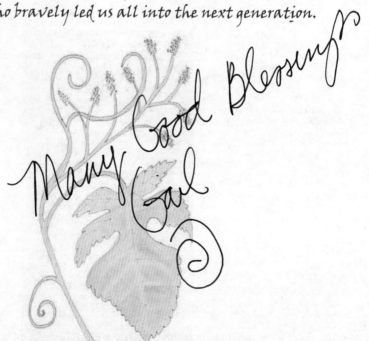

*Many Good Blessings
Gail*

TABLE OF CONTENTS

PART 1

Preface

Introduction

In the Beginning

The Land of Milk and Honey

The Goddess Religion

She Who Holds the Reins of Kings

Divine Serpent Lady

Sacred Trees

The Cumaean Sybil

The Prince of Peace

PART 2

Finding Mary

Our Wild Hearts and Mary

Reclamation

The Mary Garden

The Angelic Psalter

How to Pray the Rosary

The 20 Mysteries of the Rosary

The Joyful Mysteries

The Luminous Mysteries

The Sorrowful Mysteries

The Glorious Mysteries

PART 3

Teachings of the Herbs, Flowers and Trees of the Mysteries

Our Lady's Florilegia ~ The Rosary Garden

Joyful Mystery plants – Garlic, Onions, Leeks, Marjoram, Rosemary, Sage, Chamomile, Poppies, Figs

Luminous Mystery plants – Grains, Grapes and fermented foods and drinks, Mustard family plants.

Sorrowful Mystery plants – The Olive Tree, St. John's wort, Aloe vera, Passionflower

Glorious Mystery plants – The Rose family fruits, berries and flowers

She is the Star of the Sea – Seaweeds

Ode to Maria

Litany of Loreto

Epilogue – The Hearth Fire, Hestia's Gift

Acknowledgements and Thanks

Bibliography

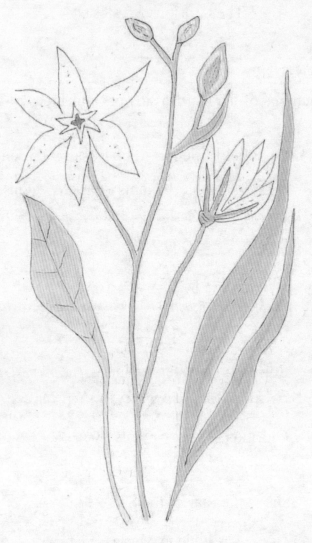

Preface

This delightful book leads us down the worn stone cobbles of Monte San Giacomo. We meet the author's friends and neighbors whose daily lives are rooted deeply in the rich soil of their gardens, even as their faith in the Madonna carries spirits aloft. The rhythms of the local planting cycles and rites of worship cultivate deeply the living of each day.

Gail Faith Edwards provides a fascinating glimpse into the ancient roots of the worship of the Mother Goddess, dating back to 35 millennia and expressed through many of the archetypal Heroines: Hera, Sybil, Venus, Eve and Mother Mary. One branch of this spiritual tradition finds the sacred Earth Goddess in the roots of fruit-bearing trees, as well as elm, sycamore and willow.

The author's sojourn evokes musings from my own journeys, during which I have trod the timeworn paths of my ancestral paternal village of Pietravairano in the Campania region of Italy, only to enter the door of the church that was blessed by the town's *Patrono*, Saint Eraclio. I have traveled with Earth stewards from Egypt, Jordan and Lebanon and walked among the wild herbs with devoted students of nature in Israel and Palestine. By moonlight, I meandered the vibrant streets of a Druze village set like a jewel on a hilltop in the Carmel Cost region of Israel, after breaking bread with a family whose lives are—as were those of their ancestors—steeped in the use of herbs for food, worship and medicine.

Culinary traditions grow out of a rich milieu defined by culture, faith and the herbs that grow in everyone's home region. In this present book, the Blessed Mother Mary, and the devotions of the rosary, form the nexus of a spiritual journey into the heart of herbalism. On these pages the well-fingered rosary beads, and their associated prayers, gradually accrue to honor the 20 mysteries of faith in Mary and Jesus.

This book takes the reader on a unique journey, from the realm of the Earth Goddess to the precepts of faith in Mother Mary. It is a story simultaneously enlightened by humanity's benevolence and darkened by our lapses into ignorance and violence born of fear.

Herein, herbal traditions are turned endearingly in the author's hands and contemplated as the beads of devotion. Believers in the Madonna, and peoples of all faiths, will discover a compendium of loving kindness, of spiritual and physical enrichment through the practices and teachings outlined here.

In "The Rosary Garden" Gail Faith Edwards tells of the herbs and other plants associated with each mystery of the Rosary. She shares the folklore of these plants and explains their botanical properties and practical uses for food and medicine. Through stories, recipes and plant lore—all of which are grounded in a thorough knowledge of botany and nutrition—this rich storehouse of wisdom reveals that herbs are a gift from God to nourish our entire beings.

Through the Wild Heart of Mary is food for body, mind and spirit. To harvest among these pages is to watch the scales of a bud unfold. The deeper layers of meaning become more pleasing when they are savored like the subtle yet complex tastes and aromas of a good basil.

Michael J. Caduto, author *Everyday Herbs in Spiritual Life: A Guide to Many Practices* (SkyLight Paths).

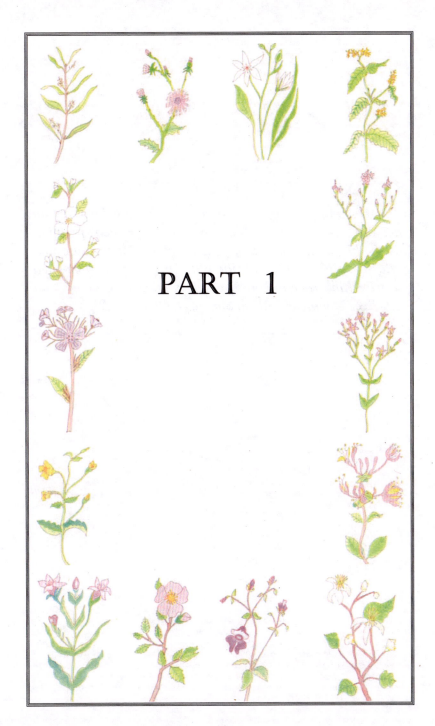

PART 1

"In the landscape of each and every human imagination lies one special place. Our inner compass keeps pointing us to this spot, which is magnetic, mysterious, exotic and alluring. It is to this specific place that we are compelled to travel in order to know ourselves and, in so doing, call our lives complete." Alvah Simon, North to the Night

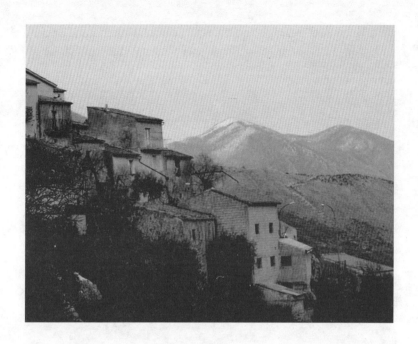

INTRODUCTION

High up in the Apennine Mountains of Southern Italy, set like a rose quartz jewel at the foot of Mount Cervati, lies the ancient village of Monte San Giacomo. Around it are 13 other villages, all of them with roots reaching back into Neolithic times, all of them climbing up into the mountains around the Valley of Diana, a lush, rich, fertile plain.

This is my ancestral home, the place where my grandmother was born, and hers before her, going back for many thousands of years. This is where my ancestors are buried. The place where their spirits still live strong and I can feel and commune with them.

The women here carry heavy loads on their heads, they run up the mountainsides herding goats well into their seventies and eighties, and lovingly tend their olive trees and gardens. Men shepherd flocks of sheep, lead horses loaded with firewood through the narrow cobblestone passageways and congregate at the local café every afternoon at 3 o'clock.

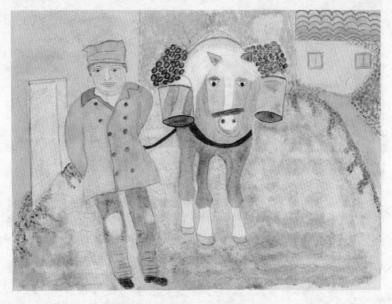

It often seems that time has stood still here, that the village is magically suspended in a timeless space. But then you notice that the kids all hold a cell phone to the side of their heads and wear the latest fashions.

The young men race their Alfa Romeo's up the road that winds into the village from the valley below and everyone is hip to the latest hip hop recording. It is a culture in perennial transition, the old residing comfortably with the new.

Our village is named after Saint James the Apostle, and was built between the 8th and 9th centuries. The main church, located in the central piazza, also bears the saint's name. (We have seven churches here in this village of 1,500.)

Sant Anna, mother of Mary and grandmother of Jesus, is the beloved patroness of our people. A beautiful and ancient shrine in her honor sits at the top of the village, near a running spring. We celebrate the feast of St. Ann every year during the middle of July. The highlight of her *festa* is a procession, during which the women carry the statue of St. Ann on a platform all the way up the hill from the village to the her shrine up above.

The Madonna is dearly loved and venerated, with almost constant novenas celebrated in her many names and in honor of her different attributes. The Immaculate Heart Of Mary, Our Lady of Perpetual Help, Our Lady of Fatima, Our Lady of Lourdes, Our Lady of Mount Carmel, Our Lady of Pompeii, Madonna de l'Neve (Our Lady of the Snow), Madonna dei Ceri, Our Lady of the Assumption and so on.

Any walk through the village or up onto the mountain presents many opportunities to enjoy well tended shrines erected by people in honor of Mary or one of the other patron saints. Inside the shrine, beside the likeness, or statue, will be flowers and candles, always kept lit.

The holy family has a real living presence here. The names of Jesus, Mary and Joseph are spoken often and always with great love and reverence. The San Giacomese people are exceptionally devout, and the spirituality that permeates life here is their common and outstanding characteristic.

The Catholic Church of *Sant Giacomo* is the heart of life in our village. Everyday life revolves around the Catholic liturgical calendar, and there is always another saint, or season, to be celebrated.

The church bells ring every fifteen minutes and can be heard throughout the village. There are several styles of rings, each having a specific meaning, such as a funeral today, a call to vespers in the evening, or the Sunday morning wakeup call. Since medieval times the church bells have served as a form of communication within the village and among its inhabitants.

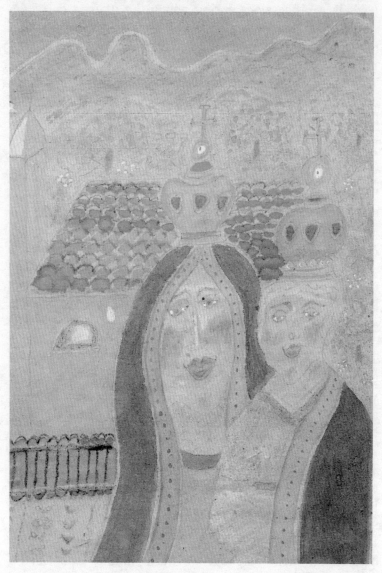

My grandmother, Maria Giuseppa, left Monte San Giacomo to come to America as a young girl of twenty, in 1905. She brought with her the deep sense of spirituality with which she had been raised, in particular a love for and devotion to the Blessed Mother. This love and veneration was passed on to her children: my mother, five aunts and two uncles, all of whom nurtured a love of Mary throughout their lives.

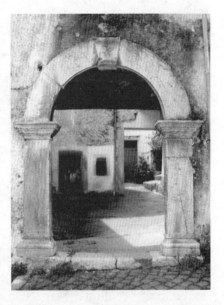

After the death of my mother, returning to my ancestral roots, learning the language of my people, and especially the prayers as they are spoken in our native dialect became very important to me. In an effort to learn more about our original homeland and culture, my daughters and I visited Monte San Giacomo one November for three weeks. We loved it! We returned for several extended stays and now have a little place of our own in the village. Fortunately for us, we found a house in a lovely courtyard next to Lisa Carmella.

Every afternoon, around the time the four o'clock church bells ring, my sweet neighbor Carmella knocks on my door and calls out to me in her delightful sing-song tone, "*Signora*..." When I open the door she is standing there with a big smile on her face. She will be dressed in her gardening clothes: a blue cotton coat, her head wrapped in a blue scarf and a pair of tennis sneakers on her feet.

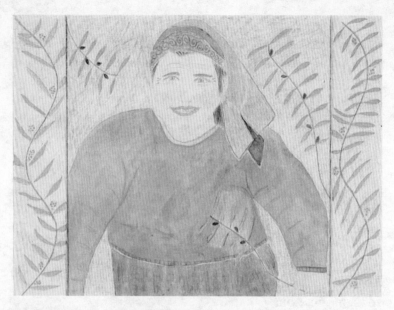

Carmella is a tireless gardener who works from morning until late afternoon tilling her soil and tending to plants and animals. She asks me if I will go to the rosary and mass with her *sta sera* (this evening). I almost always say yes and then promptly at quarter to five she is back knocking on the door, all cleaned up and dressed in her "going to church clothes." Carmella kindly offers me her arm and we walk across the cobblestone courtyard to Maria's house and call at her door. Maria usually comes right out, toting her elegant black cane with its fancy brass handle. Together the three of us walk down via napoli toward the Sant Giacomo *chiesa* (church.)

As we approach we see other women coming toward the church from every possible direction, down all the little narrow passageways leading into the piazza and toward the beautiful yellow church with the great wooden doors. Most of them, though not all, are elders. Some walk with the help of a walking stick, many are dressed from head to toe in black. Widows here in southern Italy wear black for the rest of their lives after the death of their *morito* (husband.)

These women dressed in black flood the side alleys and cobblestone streets of our village just before five o'clock. They walk in groups of twos and threes. In *Italia* people do things together, rarely alone. And since one never passes anyone without issuing a greeting of some sort, there are a lot of heads nodding and *buona seras* (good evening) said on the way into the church.

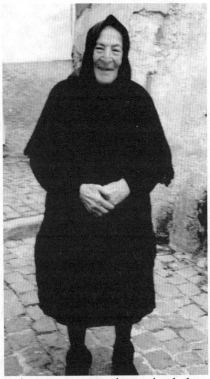

I cannot help but sense, and call attention to, the profound timelessness of this activity. For at least the past one thousand years the women of my village have come together at the end of every day for evening prayers. (Most likely this has gone on for many thousands of years, for even in pre-Christian times people regularly gathered for prayer at the centrally located temple.)

No matter what their day has brought to them, whether heartache or joy, no matter how tired they are, they walk to the church in the evening with their neighbors and lay it all at the feet of their beloved *Maria* and her son *Gesu*. They make a daily offering. They say the rosary together. They sit with their community, candle flames blazing, celebratory songs and prayers on their lips. It takes one hour of their day. They seem to give it so gladly.

Once inside the church we go directly to the water fountain, where we dip our fingers into the holy water and bless ourselves by making the sign of the cross. We each genuflect before entering our pew. Maria, Carmella and I sit shoulder to shoulder in the same pew every night. We get comfortable and take out our rosaries while the church fills up. I notice the red candles on either side of the altar are lit, and flames are rising and spiraling in groups before the statues of Sant Giacomo, Mary and Sant Lucia. The feeling inside the church is alive and vibrant.

We listen to devotional music for a short while until the rosary begins. I feel so at ease here in the church of Sant Giacomo. I feel at home and surrounded by love. I am thankful to be offering my prayers in this little church where my ancestors have been baptized and welcomed into their faith, received communion, were married, and put to rest for many centuries. I am meditating on these ancestors, and feeling joined in communion with them, and with this soulful group of women who surround me here now. A distinctive voice calls out. *Nel nome del Padre e del Figliuolo e della Spirito Santo*...And the rosary begins.

All of us are entranced in the chanting of the rosary prayers, all of us fingering our well-worn beads. The sound of all the women's voices, and those of a few men who stay in the back of the church, all intoning these familiar and deeply loved prayers out loud, in unison, is deeply nourishing. *Ave Maria, piena di grazia*...the leader's voice is clear, resonant, ringing out. *Santa Maria, Madre de Dio*...we respond. The many voices are lilting, rhythmic, plaintive. They build upon each other. The sound fills the church. The leader calls out the contemplation of the first Joyful Mystery. *La annunciazione dell'Angela a Maria Vergine...Gloria al Padre, e al Figliuolo e allo Spirito Santo...* The prayers resound from the stone walls, from the vaulted ceiling, from the marble floors.

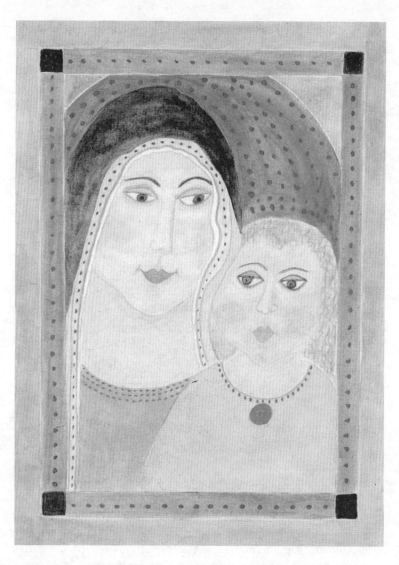

When the rosary is done, we kneel for the Salve Regina. *Hail Holy Queen, Madre di misericordia, our life our sweetness and our hope*...Is there any sweeter prayer known in all the world than this? *Turn then, most gracious advocate, your eyes of mercy toward us*...and then we chant the entire Litany of Loredo, the long call and response in praise of the Blessed Mother, Mary.

Mother of the Church, pray for us, Mother of Grace, pray for us, Mother of Good Counsel, pray for us, Virgin Most Prudent, Mirror of Justice, Seat of Wisdom, Cause of our Joy, Temple of the Holy Spirit, Mystical Rose, Gate of Heaven, Morning Star, Queen of Angels, Queen of the Most Holy Rosary, Queen of the Family, Queen of Peace…Soon we are saying, *so that we who meditate on these mysteries of the most holy Rosary of the Blessed Virgin Mary, may both imitate what they contain and attain to what they promise…through Christ our Lord. Amen.*

For a few minutes we sit in a lovely silence. The church has filled now with people who have come to attend the evening mass. The organ starts and we all stand as the priest comes onto the altar and mass begins. Padre usually keeps the mass short and sweet in the evenings, with communion and the passing of the Peace the main events. During the passing of the Peace, we warmly shake hands, saying *Pace* (Peace), with the women around us, those who share the same pew, those in front of us, the women behind us, and those across the aisle. It is wonderful looking into the eyes and smiling faces of each of the women while shaking hands with them. My voice has been joined with their voices in prayer, my heart is joined to their hearts in love and recognition. There is a sense of intimacy here, of familiarity. A sense of community and shared purpose.

The communion song begins and we process out of our pews, lining up to receive communion. Most of the elder women here are amazingly strong and vibrant. There is a lively spring in their step. Some among us are quite old and move much more slowly. All of them worked alongside their parents and other family members as young children, each of them walking for two hours every morning up the mountain where the farms are, working all day, and then carrying a bundle of firewood, potatoes or whatever they could, on their heads, back to the village below after the day's work was done. Despite the poverty and hardships they endured there is no bitterness in the telling of these tales. As a people, the San Giacomese possess a serenity, a nobility, built on a lifetime of working closely with the land and cultivating a deep sense of wonder and spirituality that is closely linked with the seasonal procession. They actively participate in the cyclical celebrations of the Catholic Church as an entire community, and these celebrations are intimately tied with the seasonal changes of the earth. The peace, calm, dignity and love that issue from living in such a way is clearly evident on their individual faces as they process down the aisle and back from communion.

The mass comes to an end, always with a song. There is a lot of singing during mass at the Sant Giacomo church. *Ave Maria,* in any number of forms, is always one of the highlights, *Alleluia* is another. We sit for a short while after the song ends, each in our own thoughts and prayers, then slowly file out of the church.

Carmella, Maria and I leave through the side door, where I love to stop and gaze for a few moments at the beautiful fresco of Jesus in a garden surrounded by angels that adorns the wall behind the altar, before going down the one step and out into the cobblestone piazza.

Once back outside, we head home in the same small groups in which we came. The women's talk is animated as we head up via napoli toward our homes. They chat happily, all the while exchanging the gossip and news of the day. I have noticed that not much happens in the village that these women do not know about. They make it their business to keep up with what is going on around them. For instance, when greeting each other on the street, they rarely ask "How you are doing?" Instead they ask "*Where* are you going?" They want to know what you are up to!

We turn onto the little passageway that leads to Maria's house and then into the courtyard where Carmella and I both live. My sweet neighbor then walks me directly to my door, waits until it is opened, and we say *buona notte,* "good night." So ends our daily evening ritual. One I have come to anticipate with joy, feel deeply nourished by and for which I am profoundly grateful

Back inside our little house, I warm myself in front of the fireplace and savor this peaceful, centered space. Soon my teenage daughter Belle will be home, we'll be listening to Ben Harper and getting dinner together, maybe enjoying a game of 500 Rummy afterward. But right now I can't help reflect on the implications and fruits of a daily hour spent in communal prayer. Or, as Pope John Paul II put it, this daily hour spent praying the rosary in *"contemplation of the face of Christ with the eyes and heart of Mary."*

This does seem to be the crux of the whole thing. It is the contemplation of Christ *with the eyes and heart of Mary* that gives the rosary and its 20 mysteries such depth of meaning. Not only for the individual, but also for the community as a whole.

For among these people, with whom recitation of the rosary and participation in the mass that follows is very much a part of daily life, long healthy vibrant lives do seem to be the norm. The village is a peaceful place to live, and the people here treat each other with love, kindness and exceptional generosity.

I wonder how much of their well-being is due to the practice of the evening rosary and communion, the singing and hand shaking, their vibrant love of Jesus, Mary, Joseph and all the saints, and the regularly experienced sense of reverence, joy and awe.

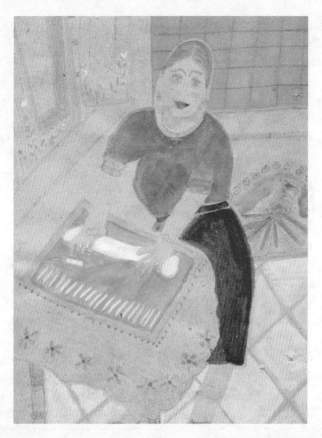

And how much is due to their earth-honoring lifestyle, which includes plenty of physical activity, fresh air, pure water and a simple diet of olive oil, fermented cheese and meats, fresh and preserved fruits, vegetables, wine, *pane* (bread) and pasta.

I've concluded that it is the combination of working closely with the land, eating and enjoying what is provided in each season, and regularly giving "thanks and praise" that has so ennobled the people of my ancestral village. I've come to appreciate their time-honored traditional ways as essential for grounding a strong foundation in physical as well as spiritual health and well-being. It is the simple wisdom of good living that they have accrued through the centuries.

I believe that we can best understand ancient culture, materials, symbols and practices in the context of the living people still inhabiting the same land and practicing the same rites as their ancestors. I feel deeply grateful to have been led to live among my native people, to learn from them and to participate with them in our collective cultural and religious celebrations still pulsing with vibrancy through the rhythm of their daily lives. I fear that the beautiful elder women of my village may be among the last to live this uncomplicated Neolithic life-style of theirs. The world, and the village, is changing so fast.

As a community herbalist, and now a grandmother, with a life-long passion for healing and teaching, I feel a strong and compelling urge to share the simple and ancient ways I've learned from my beloved "old lady friends" of Monte San Giacomo. I hope that you will receive this work as a small portion of the great body of wisdom accumulated by the indigenous people of the Apennine Mountains of Southern Italia, the descendants of the original *Lucani,* the Italic tribes who lived between the mountain peaks and the Tyrrhenian Sea for ages. I see my role in sharing what I've learned from my people, and through the participatory consciousness of our communal prayer and procession, as a sacred trust.

My purpose in writing this book is to share with you what I believe to be our common spiritual and cultural history as human beings on this planet. I want to bring to your awareness the power of the rosary as a way of prayer and meditation, and as a potent tool for grounding peace. It is essential now that we learn to broaden our capacity to both experience and extend compassion, empathy and love to all life on this earth we inhabit. To this end we will discuss the importance of developing what I refer to as our *wild hearts* and of connecting on a deep, personal level with the wild heart of Mary.

I will be sharing a few simple, time honored prayers as well as information about traditional herbs and foods that will provide us with an excellent foundation of health, not only for the body, but for strong, healthy minds and spirits too.

I am going to share Biblical stories with you also. The twenty mysteries of the rosary will provide us with the framework of our explorations here. As we will see, these ancient mystery stories have roots that penetrate deep into our common ancestral soil, into the very stuff of which we are all made. Meditation on these sacred tales brings us into communion with our primordial spiritual inheritance, connects us to our remote past, yet brings us firmly into the present moment where we can act to change an uncertain future, for the sake of all generations yet to be born on our beloved Mother Earth.

Sacred art approaches the inexpressible in ways much more powerfully evocative than mere words and text. Because we can perhaps best comprehend the totality of the sacred whole through such nonlinguistic means as symbol, color, line and form, I've included a rich assortment of imagery, including original watercolors and photographs throughout these pages. In so doing I hope to stimulate a balance between your right and left brain modes of perception and thereby enrich your experience here.

May the information you find within these pages be of benefit to you, and through you, to the entire world.

May all the world know peace and joy.

Gail Faith Edwards
March 18, 2009

To grasp the unfathomable depth of the mysteries of the rosary, we need to step all the way back in time to the beginning, for it is to the very beginning of human life and culture that we trace the roots of these spiritual stories. What follows is an overview of human history as I understand it.

IN THE BEGINNING

Our earliest human ancestors most likely lived as long ago as three million years. Fossils recently uncovered in Kenya of two different species of humans, *Homo habilis* and *H. erectus,* indicate they lived in Africa side by side for more than half a million years, roughly 1.5 million years ago.

H. habilis is thought to be the first species of the *Homo* genus to appear. Despite the fact that their cranial capacity was less than half that of modern humans, their remains are often accompanied by primitive stone tools.

A hallmark of *Homo erectus* is a distinctive teardrop-shaped stone hand axe. These implements, found at Olduvai Gorge, in northern Tanzania, one of the most important prehistoric sites in the world, were made by human hands 1.4 million years ago.

The first *Homo neanderthalensis* appeared in Europe as early as 350,000 years ago. New radiocarbon dating suggests that Neanderthals still existed in central Europe 28,000 years ago, indicating that they coexisted in central Europe with *H. sapiens* for perhaps as long as 15,000 years. These recent findings may compel scientists to rethink theories of Neanderthal extinction, intelligence and contributions to the human gene pool. Though many scholars would argue against it, these findings support the idea that there may have been a fair amount of genetic exchange between Neanderthals and modern humans.

Neanderthals buried their dead in groups, usually in a sleeping position. Analysis of fossil pollen associated with these burials suggests that the bodies were covered with shrubs and sprinkled with bachelor buttons and hollyhock flowers. They practiced tool-making and hunting and left artifacts, such as burials of cave bear skulls, that seem to indicate the practice of religious ritual.

Scientists believe we modern humans, *Homo sapiens,* arose somewhere between 100,000 and 400,000 years ago. Paleoanthropologists are still debating our origins. What we do know is that a morphologically diverse group of humans inhabited the Old World 100,000 years ago. *Homo sapiens* lived in Africa and the Southern Mediterranean, *Homo erectus* had moved into Asia, and northern and central Europe was home to *Homo neanderthalensis.*

This diversity vanished sometime between 35,000 to 50,000 years ago. By that time humans everywhere had evolved into the anatomically modern form of *Homo sapiens.*

Just how this transformation occurred is not well understood. Some scientists think that a biological change brought about by mutations played a key role in the emergence of behaviorally modern humans. This biologically based explanation implies that a major neural reorganization of the brain resulted in a significant enhancement in the manner in which the brain processed information. Other scientists posit a small group of perhaps 10,000 *Homo sapiens* migrating north out of Africa 100,000 years ago and spreading across the globe.

Our *Homo sapiens* ancestors of the Paleolithic Age were quintessentially modern in both their appearance and behavior. Technological ingenuity, intricate social formations, and ideological complexity are a hallmark of the Paleolithic peoples and significant innovations in human culture are seen during this time. It is during the later stages of the Upper Paleolithic, about 35,000 years ago, that the first art we know of appears. However, it is art of the highest refinement. According to scholars, by this time in our collective human history, art had already been evolving for thousands of years. There are brilliant artists among us now.

Ancient art is among the most magnificent art that has ever been made by human hands. More than 25,000 years ago the Venus of Willendorf was made in Austria. One of the earliest images of the female body we know of, she stands just over 4 ½ inches high and was found on the Danube river.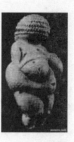

The so called "Painted Gallery" of Chauvet, in southern France is considered to be the pinnacle of Paleolithic cave art. Perhaps most stunning for the sheer number of paintings of now extinct animals, red ochre hands, and other abstract designs covering the walls, it goes back to 16,500 B.C. These red, and sometimes red and black, hands painted around entrances to caves appear continuously throughout the Paleolithic from 20,000 - 10,000 B.C. They are believed to possess energizing and healing powers, to promise abundance and symbolize the protective touch of the Goddess.

A prehistoric map of the night sky on the wall of this cave depicts three bright stars that are known today as the Summer Triangle.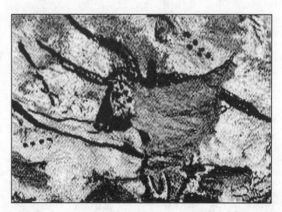

A map of the Pleiades star cluster has also been found among the Lascaux frescoes.

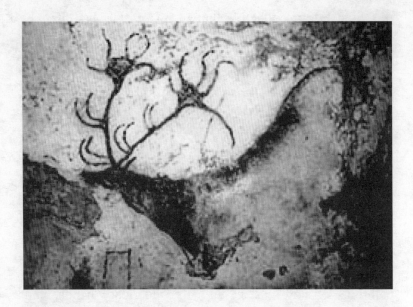

The stunning images of animals painted on cave walls, such as those at Catal Huyuk (7,000 - 5,000 B.C.) in Anatolia, which is present day Turkey, are remarkable. That the animals are in motion is unmistakable. The lines are vivid, bold and confident, the paintings skillfully executed. The power, dignity and poise of the animal are striking, yet there is subtlety here also, in the expert use of shading and the way deep emotional content is conveyed.

Countless small hand sized images beautifully drawn on stone, exquisite carvings in bone, horn and stone, the great majority of which are of the female form, are some of the innumerable artifacts uncovered throughout the Old World that attest to the artistic accomplishment and spiritual awareness of these ancient people.

Art is part of life, and ritual, ceremony, art and life are strongly bound together. These early peoples honored a Mother whose generation and cyclic changes gave birth to all and received all back into herself.

"Her worship seems to have evolved from the awe experienced by our early ancestors as they regularly observed woman's body as the source of life. Paleolithic statues celebrate the mysteries of the female: Woman's body bled painlessly in rhythm with the moon, and her body miraculously made people, then provided food for the young by making milk." Charlene Spretnak

Not only an abundance of elaborate art but also items of personal adornment are widespread and raw materials such as flint and shells are traded over distances. Burials are accompanied by ritual and include a rich assortment of grave goods. Living spaces are skillfully constructed and contain well-designed fireplaces. Some even have running water, flush toilets and bathtubs. Though many well designed tools and implements are found, there is a noticeable absence of weaponry.

My ancient southern Italian ancestors, grandmothers to the original Italic tribes that inhabited southern Italy for many thousands of years, were hunter gatherers during this time, and lived in caves or under large stone overhangs scattered throughout the Apennine Mountains.

Many of these caves were quite enormous, contained fresh water, and went into the earth in a labyrinthine maze for many miles. They could easily be, and indeed were, home to large tribes of people. The remains of human culture found in caves around our remote mountain village go back at least 60,000 years. Because of this our entire locale, one of the last truly wild and untouched wilderness areas in the world, is both a National Park and a designated UNESCO World Heritage site and will be forever protected.

"The early Italians spoke languages descending from a mother tongue called Sabellic and written in scripts modeled on Greek, Latin or Etruscan alphabets...In the

ninth century B.C. when the Romans were merely a smallish farming tribe living in huts near the Tiber, Italy was teeming with distinctive cultures, languages, and works of art and craft... By the first century B.C. though, the last traces of their political autonomy had been surrendered to the Roman Empire." Erla Zwingle, Italy Before the Romans

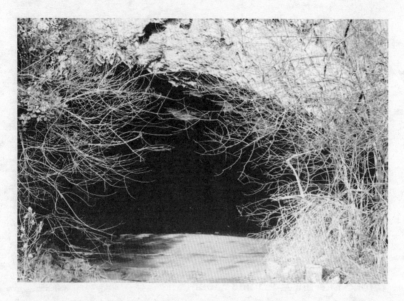

Italia today is rich in the words, customs, art and religious practices drawn from these pre-Roman Italic peoples. Their ideas, ingenuity and devotional ways are just a few of a multitude of elements that until recently were thought to originate with the Romans. Archaeological finds are now showing that in fact the Romans merely adopted them from the earlier Italic peoples.

The pre-Indo-European Italic tribes honored trinities of gods and these divinities spoke to them through the wonders of the natural world. They were clearly a Shamanic people. From their observation of the flight of birds, strikes of lightning or the peal of thunder, they derived predictions of what their future might hold. They created masterpieces of art and architecture in bone and stone. Their words, which they considered sacred, murmur to us across the centuries: *maatir,* mother; *puklum,* son... Their images do too.

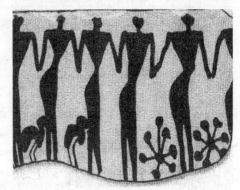

When did our early Mediterranean and Old World mothers first start to paint the dancing and life-like figures holding hands alongside plants and birds found on 35,000-year-old pottery shards?

These images tell of a people who were celebrating being in peaceful community with all other living beings. *A people for whom not only words but all of life was held sacred.*

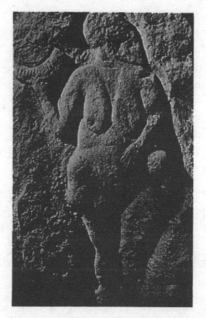

When did women first carve lines on bone to mark their menstrual flow, the phases of the moon or the rising of stars? Some of the earliest artifacts are menstrual calendars: animal bones and horns notched with lunar cycles. Our ancient mothers kept these lunar - menstrual calendars at least 20,000 years ago. They observed the moon phases in relation to the positions of stars and planets using their own synchronized menstrual cycles as the biological norm. The notational system they used evolved into a refined system of mathematics and a sophisticated science that informed their daily lives and seasonal rituals.

They developed and kept highly evolved records of night time sky patterns and left us the remains of their study. Their ingenuity and astute observational skills gave birth to writing, complex calendars, astronomy and astrology.

The archaeological record plainly shows that our Paleolithic ancestors were a Shamanic people who revered the Feminine, were keenly in touch with the energies of their bodies, the earth, the heavens, the movements of the stars, planets and wild animals, the turning of the seasons and the returning of plants and birds. They were deeply in tune with and knowledgeable about the cosmos and each other and possessed language abilities equivalent to our own.

The Paleolithic gradually became the Neolithic period over many thousands of years. By 8,000 B.C. in the Near East and southern Mediterranean areas people were peacefully domesticating animals, cultivating grains and inhabiting permanent village communities. Pottery, weaving, spinning, and architecture using masonry, wood and stone, all were widespread and in common use by this time.

When the Iceman, or "Otzi," was found in the Italian Alps near the border with Austria several years ago, he conveyed quite a bit of information about the Neolithic period for a silent, albeit well preserved, 5,000-year-old mummy.

The shoes he was wearing were sturdy and well made, with thick bear skin soles. His clothing was expertly woven of natural materials and sewn with such skill that it would be hard to duplicate in today's world. Among the items he carried with him were a finely made copper axe, polypore mushrooms and tinder for starting a fire. When scientists examined a tiny portion of the remains in his intestines, they found he had been eating barley and an early cultivar of wheat known as einkorn.

Both these grains were being cultivated in Neolithic settlements south of the Alps by 5,000 to 8,000 years ago, and bread was being baked in stone ovens. Minuscule remains of the charcoal on the bread Otzi had eaten were also detected.

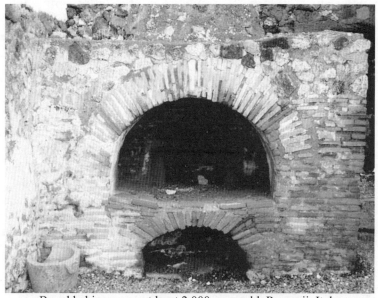
Bread baking oven, at least 2,000 years old, Pompeii, Italy

There are farmers, gardeners and shepherds now. Finely crafted tools indicate that people are tilling the earth, planting and harvesting. The domestication of animals developed around this same time. The ongoing refinement of technique, craftsmanship and beauty of shape, color and form continues to be evident in tools and implements of the Neolithic.

Gold, copper and bronze are known and used now. An infinite variety of clay pots are beautifully painted with what had long been considered "abstract ornamental patterns," but revealed by archaeologist Marija Gimbutas to be a rich and vibrant written language which she referred to as the "Language of the Goddess."

It is largely because of the brilliant, diligent and intuitive work of Marija Gimbutus, that we have as accurate a picture as we do of the Neolithic Old World people and culture. Combining her knowledge of 22 languages with extensive archaeological evidence, as well as cross-cultural mythology, folklore and symbolic interpretation, Gimbutas revealed the existence of a widespread prehistoric culture centered on the Goddess as life giver and sustainer, as well as death-wielder. In her books, such as *The Language of the Goddess* and others, Gimbutas clearly explains the archaeological evidence and shows how the venerated position of the Goddess in the lives of these early people changed with the incursions by Kurgan groups into their areas (4,300-2,800 B.C.) She describes how the Old World moved from a matrilineal culture based on loyalty to the clan to a patrilineal society based on hierarchy over the ensuing centuries.

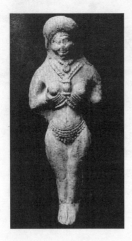

The Near East was the cradle of civilization and culture slowly spread across the Mediterranean into southern Europe. In 7,000 B.C. Jericho, in Mesopotamia, was a settled community of neat stone houses with plaster floors, clay ovens and rectangular shrines in every home. The town was well fortified, protected by walls and towers of strong masonry construction.

Many small clay figurines with hands raised to their breasts have been uncovered here. They resemble other figurines widely distributed throughout the Near East. Historic documents refer to this Goddess as the *Queen of Heaven*.

The ancient Sumerians were an innovative and creative people who arrived in southern Mesopotamia sometime around 4,000 B.C. from Persia. Over the next thousand years they created a number of city-states and developed a unique form of cuneiform writing on clay tablets. They built stone houses around a large sacred area that contained the shrines and temple and also workshops, storehouses, and residential buildings inhabited by the priestesses who served the temple. The temple was placed at the very center of this sacred area on a raised platform indicating the leading role it played in the life of the community.

Sumerian cuneiform tablets written in 2,600 B.C. describe their dietary staples; garlic, grains, legumes, root vegetables, leafy greens, cucumbers and a variety of fish.

The Sumerians were practicing astrology 5,000 years ago. Their ancient legends say that we are fashioned out of clay by a great Mother Goddess, Nammu, whose name means *"sea"* and the *"mother who gave birth to both heaven and earth."* Later, and in other cultures, this ancient mother is known as Nina, Nanshe, Ninmah, Ninkasi and Ningal.

She is Nana, the Oldest One.
Serpent Goddess of the Oracles
Mistress of Decrees, Interpreter of Dreams.
It is she who assigns the destinies of life.
She is Nidaba, Goddess of Wisdom
Holy Cobra, Ancient Scribe.
She teaches the knowledge of the written word
and writes all our deeds upon the leaves
of the Tree of Life.

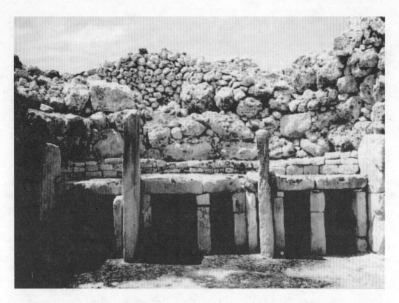

Across the Mediterranean, on the island of Malta, around this same time, people were building megalithic temples that still stand. The oldest standing stone structures on earth, these temples were built from 4,000 to 2,500 B.C. and predate both Stonehenge and the Pyramids.

These people are thought to have crossed the sea from Sicily and arrived on the Maltese Islands more than 7,000 years ago. They were farmers and shepherds who grew grains and kept domesticated animals. They worshipped a Mother Goddess whose likeness is found throughout the Mediterranean.

Life during the Neolithic period was essentially rural, peaceful and self sufficient. I think it must have been a lot like our Italian village is today.. Social relationships were loosely woven associations between family, clans and tribe. Concerns centered around village life, and most villages were built around a sacred center. Well defined customs and traditions, which had evolved over the millennia and were unique to each place, were passed on through the generations orally, *without the aid of written records.*

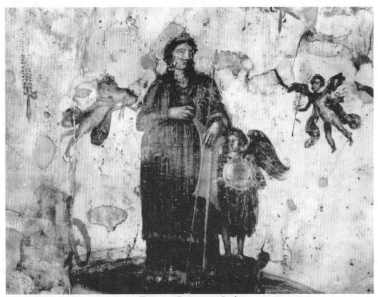

Fresco, Pompeii, Italy

My sense is that "without the aid of written records" is somehow important. These were a pre-literate people. They did not use the word to rule, to claim superiority, to intimidate, to create a separate, learned class or to gain knowledge to use as power over others.

Many of the elder women in our village do not read or write. Yet they recite all the chants and prayers and sing all the alternating songs of the Catholic liturgy, hundreds of them, some quite long, all by heart and with great feeling. And I wish you could see how they work with the earth. With such brilliance do they know when to plant and when to harvest, when to prune and what to do with what they've gathered. Raising animals for milk and meat is also something they do with tenderhearted care and loving attention.

These agricultural tasks are aligned with the seasonal celebrations of the church, and so these women's lives are intimately connected with earth and spirit throughout the year. My neighbor Carmella was taught by her mother that the day to plant the first lettuce seeds of the season is on the Feast of the Presentation, February 1, also known as Candlemas Day. Sure enough, true to her mother, Carmella plants her lettuce seeds on that day every year.

Traditional, earth-based peoples pay attention to the dynamics of the natural world around them. They are acutely aware of the dramas, rhythms and presence of a place and feel a profound connection to and love for it. Throughout time one's sense of place has been a refuge. It has offered strength and stability as well as ethnic identity.

I believe that this ethnic identity, the culture, language, habits and customs of a people who have evolved over thousands of years of living in one place, is an immensely precious thing. It is a rich and radiant pool of wisdom from which we all can learn. Our individual ethnic identities must be honored, celebrated, protected and generously shared rather than sanitized or eliminated as is the trend in the current movement toward homogenization and globalization.

The elders of our village know the intricate family histories, by marriage as well as by blood, of all the other people in the village, for generations. So much so that they recognized and welcomed my children and I as *San Giacomese,* even though my grandmother left the village 99 years, practically to the day, before we arrived!

I think of the magnanimous love and compassion they all have in their hearts and express without constraint. It is just bursting out of them, this love. I am in awe of their incredible beauty, knowledge, wisdom and unique way of perceiving and being in the world. These fruits of a life well lived the old ones here exude - many of them without knowing how to read or write a single word.

Images speak louder and clearer than words. In the main square, or *casale*, the first thing one sees when entering our village is a beautiful mosaic of St. Joseph holding the baby Jesus. Another beloved patron of our village is St. Rocco, always seen with a tiny dog at his side.

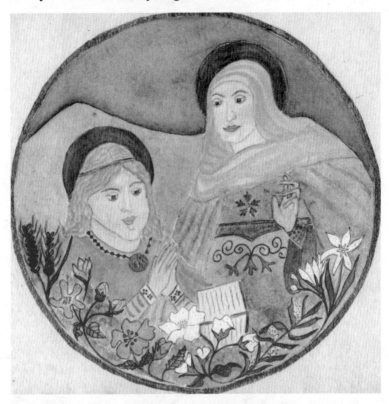

The shrine of St. Anna stands at the top of a hill, not far from the stone remains of the first settlers here. A vibrant spring still flows behind her shrine. St. Anna is our all present *Nona,* protector and instructor. She is usually depicted viewing a book with her adolescent daughter Mary. Next to the shrine of St. Anna stands the shrine of St. Antonio, patron of orphans and little children. In the middle of January the children of our village go door to door collecting firewood from which they will make a large bonfire to celebrate the life and work of this saint.

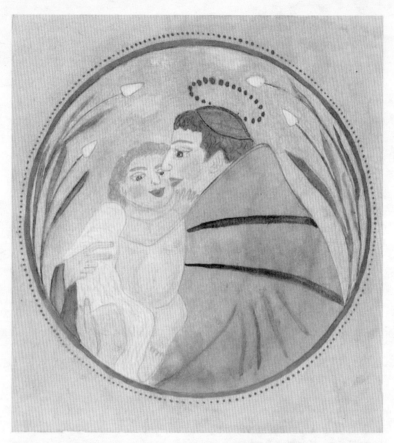

Beautiful paintings, mosaics, sculptures and shrines of the Madonna and Child are everywhere. These images serve as pictorial teachers. They let the boys and men in our village know that it is in their nature to be nurturing and kind; it is their duty to look out for and protect those in need, including the many stray dogs and cats that freely roam our village passageways. They instruct us to respect our elders, as the transmitters of our culture, history and traditions; to love and respect our parents, because they have given us life and have cared for us. We are inspired to hold our family dear, as it is a sacred entity, a Holy Family, and this honor and respect is extended to neighbors and friends. These images inform us that we are not alone, and that our life and our interactions with all others is in essence a spiritual practice.

I see this simple yet profound culture that has been maintained and passed on through the eons as, in so many ways, far superior to the secular Western life-style we are all so familiar with.

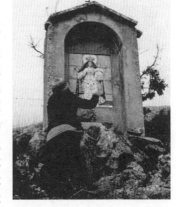

In his book *The Alphabet Vs The Goddess*, Leonard Shlain discusses the conflict between word and image. He proposes that the process of reading and writing profoundly altered the human brain, changing it from right brain dominant to left brain dominant. The right brain is associated with what we might call feminine aspects, such as intuition, holistic thinking and feeling. The left brain is more "masculine" and in charge of logical, linear thinking.

According to Shlain, this shift upset the balance between male and female, ushered in the modern era and encouraged misogynistic assumptions about women whose ancient ways and customs then fell into decline. Shlain posits that the present proliferation of images in Western culture through film, T.V., graphics and computers is now again reconfiguring the brain by stimulating right hemispheric modes of thought, thereby encouraging the reemergence of the feminine into modern culture.

Reverence for all life, especially as symbolized by the female, life-sustaining form, was widespread throughout the Neolithic period. In fact, reverence for the Mother, as embodied by the earth and all biological and cosmological processes, had been carried over from the Paleolithic.

This self fertilizing/creating-herself-Goddess is the most persistent image of these early, nonviolent cultures. For at least as far back as 35,000 years, and some say much longer, humans worshiped this Divine Mother.

The adoration of Great Mother was spread over a geographically vast area and evolved along with our human ancestors over many thousands of years. And, as Vickie Noble points out in her book *Shakti Power*, there is some evidence that reverence for the Divine Feminine may extend to the very dawn of human consciousness.

The body is a finely tuned and highly intelligent instrument, sensitive to an enormous range of subtle dynamics from which it perceives and organizes information. The earth also behaves like a living organism. It too is self-regulating, self-organizing and self-healing. Life is an interactive phenomenon with all of life adapting, interacting and affecting the rest, as in a constant feedback loop. Our ancestors perceived and revered the cyclic stages of life, death, and rebirth through women, through the earth. They were much wiser and more refined than we have previously been led to believe.

An 8,000-year-old plaque found in a shrine at Catal Huyuk depicts a couple in a loving embrace on one side and on the other the image of a mother and infant, perhaps one of the earliest *Madonnas*.

Understanding our ancestors and the origins of culture and religion in the Near East and Mediterranean opens the door to understanding the true story of our own history, spirituality and culture. We're all taught in school that Western culture begins with the Greeks, but our true story is much older than that. As we have seen, written language was in use, fine art was being created and great cities were built many centuries before the classical Greek period.

"For thousands of years before the classical myths took form and then were written down by Hesiod and Homer in the 7th century B.C., a rich oral tradition of mythmaking had existed." Charlene Spretnak

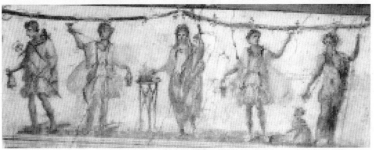

2,000-year-old fresco, Pompeii, Italy

Long before the Greeks and their gods, there was Great Goddess. There was language, art, literature and math, poetry, architecture, prophecy, divination and herstory. And, there appears to have been peace.

"The earliest law, government, medicine, agriculture, architecture, metallurgy, wheeled vehicles, ceramics, textiles and written language were initially developed in societies that worshipped the Goddess." Merlin Stone

The past is our heritage. It is our roots and our sustenance. Knowing the true story of the past brings us nourishment through the ages. This knowledge opens up doors to us, presents us with a myriad of new possibilities. It connects us to our ancestors. This nourishing connection gives us the courage and strength to act in the present. It reveals and makes very clear what needs to be done.

And we know that when we see something that needs to be done, we better get busy and do it.

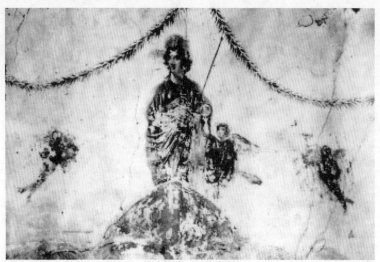
Fresco, Pompeii, Italy

A MEDITATION...

Sit down in the dark, damp cave. Feel the earth under you. Feel the warmth of the fire. Make yourself comfortable. You are at home here. You are safe. Listen for the distant waves rolling ashore onto the beach a short distance away. Hear the sweet murmur of the sea. Notice how quietly moisture moves down the walls of the cave. Hear the water dripping from the stalactites hanging from the ceiling. See how the firelight catches them as they glisten and sparkle. It is as if they are singing to you, a song of dancing light and joy. A chant starts up and you join in. Suddenly there are thousands of voices, like waves, gently rolling one upon the other. Thousands of voices, all of your extended clan is here in the cave with you and you are all singing ancient praises to the Mother. Let your voice rise up in harmony...

The waves of your lilting voices singing in veneration travel across the millennia. You each envision her in a different way. She is the sea, the rolling waves, the fish that swim and give their lives for our nourishment. She is the cave itself and the running stream within it and the crystals that hang and shimmer. She is the fire. She is the moon and the sun and the stars that shine from the sky and move across the heavens. She is the blood that flows from women to nourish the earth. She is the plants and trees that spring from the earth and all the animals upon it. She is the hills and valleys and the mountains and upon every mountain top there is a shrine to her. There are sanctuaries in her name throughout the cave and throughout the land...

She has many names, many attributes. She offers many gifts. In every small village and among every large tribe, gratitude to her plays a big part in the dynamics of daily life. Complex theological structures evolved over the millennia that included seasonal ritual dramas enacted at religious ceremonies and sacred festivals held in her honor. Many of these continue into the present day.

These rites and rituals shared the same cosmological themes but differed according to the individual customs and beliefs of people in diverse geographical areas. They coincided with the seasonal progression of the earth and were intimately tied into the rhythms of body, earth and sky. Veneration of Great Mother as wise Creator of the Universe and of all life and civilization evolved uniformly and uniquely among all these peoples.

These tribes and clans of Neolithic society were matrilineal organizations. They were peaceful tribes of earth-and-Goddess-honoring, ingenious, intelligent and highly civilized agrarian people, located throughout the entire geographic area known as the Old World. Names, social status, wealth and ownership of property were passed along through the line of the mother.

Their ancient matriarchal clan culture and the complex religious traditions that had evolved over the preceding eons, were destroyed over the ensuing centuries by waves of conquerors who came from the north in repeated attacks.

Though no one is exactly certain where the first of these northern conquerors originated, most scholars agree they were the Kurgan culture of northern Russia, nomadic hunting and fishing groups living in areas north of the Black Sea and the Caucasus. Bands known as the "battle-axe culture" also came into southern Europe and across the Near East from the northern forests and coastal areas of Europe and Denmark.

These attacks were waves of migrations and invasions that took place over a period of from one to two thousand years approximately around 4,000 to 3,000 B.C., and they continued into the historic period, approximately 2,400 B.C., which is confirmed by written accounts, records, literature and artifacts.

These aggressive, warlike people are usually referred to as Indo Europeans. In some ancient texts they are called the Aryans. Merlin Stone, author of *When God Was A Woman,* calls them the Hittites. They are described as pastoral, patriarchal, warlike and expansive.

They came riding chariots two abreast, pulled by horses, and carrying iron spears, into cultures using donkeys to pull wagons for transporting people and goods. They introduced smelting iron. Their military might had previously been unknown among the Old World peoples.

They brought with them a male storm god on a mountain top, blazing with light, fire or lightning. They presented him as intimidating and superior to the Goddess of the indigenous peoples. Their advancement through the lands of the Goddess worshiping people was marked by widespread destruction.

"The Aryans came into contact with highly civilized and already ancient forms of settled society, in comparison with they were complete and utter barbarians." Merlin Stone

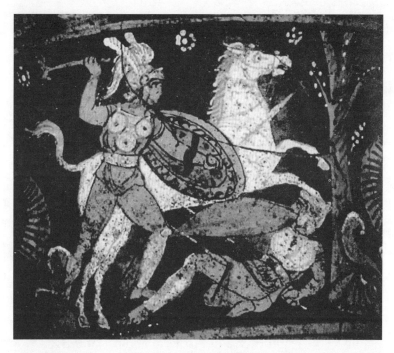

The Goddess religions assimilated the male deities into their worship and the Goddess survived as the religion of the people for thousands of years after the initial invasions.

Over the centuries of disruption, the invaders established themselves as an exclusive caste, designated the roles of royalty and leadership to themselves, and dominated the original inhabitants, who then became subservient to the invaders, or a "conquered class."

The invaders infiltrated over time by marrying the priestesses and princesses of the area and were well established throughout the Old World by the 15th century B.C.

OUR TIME LINE.

Using the genealogies given in the Old Testament to calculate, most authorities estimate the account of the Biblical creation to have taken place somewhere between 5,500 B.C. and 4,000 B.C.

The Book of Genesis sets Adam and his immediate descendants in a farming culture. Adam's task was to work and take care of the garden and to name the livestock (Gen 2:15-19). Cain worked the soil and offered the fruits of his field to the Lord. Abel offered the firstborn of his flock of sheep (Gen 4:2-4, 20).

Archaeologists trace the beginnings of plant cultivation to 10,000-7,000 B.C., with the domestication of cattle and sheep appearing soon after. So Adam, Eve, Cain and Able must have lived somewhere around this time, which was the Neolithic period. Biblical scholars date Noah, primeval ancestor of the Hebrews. at about 2,000 B.C., Abraham at about 1,800-1,500 B.C. and Moses at about 1,300 B.C.

Human culture, history and religion had already been evolving for at least 30,000 years by this time...The early Goddess figurines date to 35,000 B.C. and indicate that earth/female centered religious practice is well underway by this time.

"When compared to the religions of the Goddess in Europe and elsewhere, the Judeo-Christian tradition was "born yesterday." Charlene Spretnak, Lost Goddesses of Early Greece

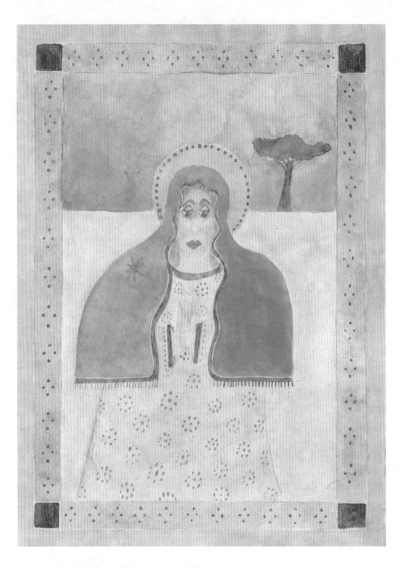

LAND OF MILK AND HONEY

The area called Canaan in the Bible, *the Land of Promise* of the Hebrews, lies at the southern tip of the region known as the Fertile Crescent and today encompasses parts of Syria, Lebanon, Palestine and Israel. Canaan is the original name of this entire area, taken from an ancestor of its early inhabitants. Palestine is the modern form of the word *Philistine*, the name of a people who settled in the southwest portion of this area. This land is often referred to as the Holy Land, as it is where Jesus lived and died. The land itself is blessed with lush meadows and fertile valleys, hills and mountains, deserts and oases, rivers and lakes. It receives plentiful rain to nourish growing plants, and enjoys mild temperatures.

In biblical times oaks, terbinths and Judas trees grew in the woodlands. "Cyclamen, rockrose, thorn apple, sage, and wormwood" also grew wild here, Vincenzina Krymow tells us in her book *Healing Plants of the Bible*. Bay laurel, carob trees, olive trees and grape vineyards all thrived around Galilee. Almond trees climbed Mount Tabor.

The Serpent Goddess, or Cobra Woman, was the widespread female deity of Canaan in ancient times. She was known as Anath, Ashtoreth, Ashtart and Asherah.

> *Asherah, Holy Queen,*
> *Mother of All Wisdom,*
> *She Who Builds.*
> *Asherah taught the people the art of carpentry*
> *and the knowledge of making bricks from clay.*

The early Semitic people honored a multi-faceted Goddess, and her attributes included fertility, sexuality, creation of life, prophecy, judgment, divine decree and guardianship, the right to rule, and concern for the oppressed and mistreated. She also embodied martial aspects such as *Goddess of Battle* and *Woman of Great Valor and Strength*.

She was the *Fruitful Mother of the Clan*, the leader in both peace and war. She was revered as the supreme divinity, honored as *"Mother of All Deities,"* and she flourished for thousands of years throughout the lands now known as the birthplace of Judaism and Christianity. Isis and Hathor were also revered here before the Hebrews arrived.

As the Israelites approached Canaan, in about 1,300-1,250 B.C., an advance envoy reported back to them that it was a *"land of milk and honey and the inhabitants were powerful and lived in fortified cities."* Numbers 13:28.

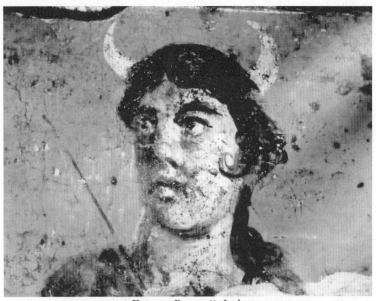

Fresco, Pompeii, Italy

The symbols, myths and ancient customs of the religion of the Goddess were the target of Hebrew aggression. The Hebrews intention, as allegedly ordered by Yahweh, was to destroy the Canaanite's altars, break down their images and cut down their sacred groves for *"thou shalt worship no other god. For the Lord whose name is jealous is a jealous god."* Exodus 34:11-16.

The Hebrews' entrance into the Promised Land was a series of bloody sieges. *"In all we took sixty cities. Then we put to death all the men, women and dependants in every city."* Deuteronomy 2:33.

In Numbers 31:17 we learn that under the leadership of Moses and Aaron, the Israelites were told to *"kill every male dependent, and kill every woman who has had intercourse with a man, but spare for yourselves every woman among them who has not had intercourse."* Their booty included *"sheep, cattle, asses and thirty two thousand girls who had no intercourse with a man." Numbers 31:32-35*

In the Battle of Ai the Hebrews killed 12,000 people in one day. According to Joshua 10:28-40, they massacred the population of the entire region, leaving no survivors, as the God of Israel had commanded. So began a violent religious persecution that in many ways, and on many levels, continues today.

Merlin Stone, in *When God Was a Woman*, quotes many passages from the Book of Genesis that record connections between Abraham and immediate descendants of the Indo-European Hittites. Among them she cites that Abraham, his wife and grandson are all buried on Hittite land. And that Abraham's two sons Jacob and Esau chose their wives from among the Hittites. Their sons also married Hittite women.

Abraham and his descendants also share the same great shining-light-on-the-mountain symbols as those of the invading Indo-Europeans. Yahweh spoke out of the fire on Mt. Horeb. This fire or light or lightning on the mountain is also associated with Moses on Mount Sinai, and later with Jesus on Mt. Tabor.

Based on her extensive research, and using her skills of deduction, Stone presents the possibility that *"The Indo European group Luvites or Luvians, may have been the original priestly Levites of the Hebrews."*

She cites their use of a separate written language, more closely resembling an ancient form of sacred hieroglyphics that contained their codex of religious laws and procedures.

Although the Levites, who were said to lead by "a day's journey ahead," may have been descendants of the Indo-Europeans, the rest of the Hebrew tribes were clearly descended from the Mediterranean Goddess-worshiping people, and they continued their ancient religious customs - not only during their time in the desert, but for many centuries after settling in the Promised Land.

Throughout the Bible there are repeated accounts of the people going back to worshiping as their ancestors had before them. In Judges 2:13 we read *"and they forsook the Lord and worshipped Baal and Ashtoreth."*

Later in Samuel 7:3-4, the people are told to *"put away the strange gods and Ashtoreth from among you..."*

According to the Bible, even the great King Solomon, 960-922 B.C., to whom the lush and lyrical Song of Solomon is attributed, worshiped Ashtoreth and other local deities. He was threatened with the loss of his kingdom for forsaking Yahweh and revering the Queen of Heaven.

The Bible reports that idols of the female deity Asherah are found on every high hill, under every green tree and alongside the altars in the temples. The tree was the universal symbol of the goddess. These Asherah (or Asherim) may have been a tree or pole perhaps carved as a statue, or they may have been sycamore fig trees which were considered in Egypt to be the "Body of the Goddess on Earth."

In Kings 17:9 we are told that *"the people of Israel did secretly against the Lord their God things that were not right. They built high places, set up pillars and asherim on every high hill and under every green tree. They served idols, made molten images of two calves (the symbol of the Goddess Hathor was a calf), they made an asherah and sold themselves to do evil in the sight of the Lord."*

The Levites declared the Hebrew mission to destroy these symbols of the Goddess religion as was commanded by Yahweh. The Levites wrote the destruction of the Divine Ancestress into their laws and set in motion the final end of the matrilineal clan system.

Deut 13:6 "If your brother or son or daughter or wife or friend suggest serving other gods, you must kill him."

PAGAN QUEEN JEZEBEL

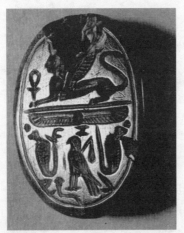

Phoenician Queen Jezebel, who lived in the 9th century B.C., is portrayed in the Bible as treacherous and evil, but her real transgression was refusing to worship Yahweh. Her royal seal indicates the pagan Queen was a powerful woman with far-reaching business dealings. Jezebel revered the Queen of Heaven, as was the way of her parents and her ancestors. King Ahab, her husband, followed her lead and erected an asherim in the temple.

That she had her own royal seal means that Queen Jezebel exerted a powerful influence on those around her, much as the Egyptian queens did. Egyptian queens were respected and potent monarchs. They played prominent roles in religion, politics and representational art.

The Hebrews, however, did not look favorably upon powerful women. Queen Jezebel was perceived as a threat and a foreign idol worshipper, accused of prostitution, murder and sorcery, and thrown from her window to be ravaged by dogs. Queen Jezebel's gruesome murder was then recorded in the Bible as a warning to other women.

After claiming her royal throne for himself, her executioner, the Hebrew hero Jehu, invited all followers of the Goddess to a gathering at the temple. When the sacred shrine was packed with her worshipers, a large band of soldiers outside were ordered to kill everyone inside the temple. Yahweh told Jehu afterward: *"Thou hast done well that which is right in mine eyes."* 11 Kings 10:18-31

The Book of Ezekiel tells us that 300 years later, in 620 B.C., there were women weeping for Tammuz at the temple in Jerusalem. The ancient mourning ceremonies of the religion of the *Queen of Heaven* were still being carried on. The women are stalwart; they will not give up the Goddess.

Although the official religion of Israel was that of Yahweh, both biblical verses and the archaeological evidence clearly shows that the cult of Baal and Astarte continued to strongly influence the people through folk customs and popular religious beliefs throughout the centuries. In fact, abundant archaeological evidence indicates that adoration of the Goddess appears to be one of the major influential factors in the development of Judaic and later Christian attitudes.

It was not until A.D. 300 that Emperor Constantine brought an end to the ancient sanctuary of Ashtoreth at Aphaca and finally suppressed her worship throughout Canaan. The following two centuries brought the final end to the last great Goddess centers, or saw their conversion into Christian churches.

"I will put an end to all her rejoicing, her feasts, her new moons, her Sabbaths and all solemn festivals." Hosea

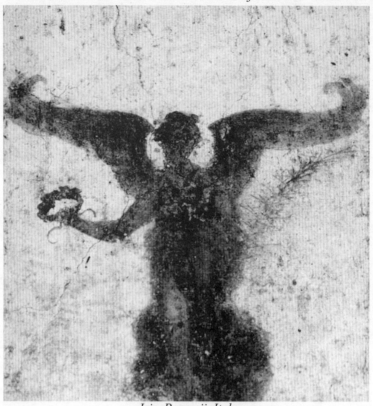

Isis, Pompeii, Italy

What was this Goddess Religion? Why did the Hebrews and Indo-Europeans want to stamp it out so badly?

The female faith was a complex theological structure, and it affected all aspects of the lives of those who worshiped the Goddess. Though, as has been seen above, the religion differed somewhat according to geographical location, many of its features were universal.

During the Neolithic period the temple was the core of the community. Records show that the temples enjoyed prosperity, that they owned much of the surrounding lands, kept herds of domesticated animals, had workshops and storehouses for food and kept the cultural and economic records of the community. The temple functioned as the central controlling offices for the public.

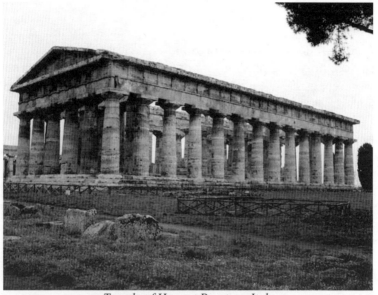

Temple of Hera at Paestum, Italy

The temple of Diana at Ephesus, built in the sixth century B.C., was one of the Seven Wonders of the ancient world. Its roof beams were made of huge cedar logs, and the entire temple covered over an acre of ground. The columns were 55 feet high and 6 feet thick at their base. It was burned to the ground in 356 B.C., on the same night, according to ancient legends, that Alexander the Great was born.

Priestesses of the Goddess provided wise counsel, prophecy and advice at her shrines. Because women are intuitive, expressive and emotional, they were considered the ideal mediums for divine revelation. The priestesses offered politically important revelations and held vital advisory positions within the community. They were highly respected and considered both wise and exceedingly knowledgeable. In fact, the priestess was perceived as the living entity of the Goddess.

"The Queen of Heaven was most reverently esteemed by the sacred women who in turn were protected by her." MS

Life, and the generation of life, was seen as divine in the Mediterranean Old World religion. Sex was considered sacred, holy and precious among these ancient peoples and was enacted within the temple, home of the divine ancestress. She was revered as the patron deity of sexual love and procreation, and sex was perceived as her gift to humanity.

Both married and single women resided within the temple complex for periods of time. They were free to come and go at will. It is recorded that women of all socio-economic groups participated in the sexual customs of the Goddess and that many were from wealthy families who engaged in extensive business dealings.

The temple women were known in their own language as "qadishtu," which literally means *sacred woman, holy woman, the undefiled, sanctified woman.* In Babylon these woman were called "Ishtaritu," or *Women of Ishtar.*

Ishtar, Queen of Heaven
Revered as Mother of the Semitic peoples along the
Euphrates and Tigris rivers.
Your images are the horned heifer and eight pointed star.
Armed with bow and arrow, you ride upon a large bird.

You are called by many names:
Guiding Light, Star of Prophecy, Mother of All,
Shepherdess of the Lands, Possessor of Life's Records,
Lady of Battle and of Victory,
Lady of Vision

Strabo, writing in Anatolia (modern day Turkey), shortly before the time of Christ, recorded the Goddess customs followed in the name of Cybele. According to him all children born to temple women were legitimate and given the names and social status of the mother. Strabo wrote that *"the unmarried mother seems to be worshiped."*

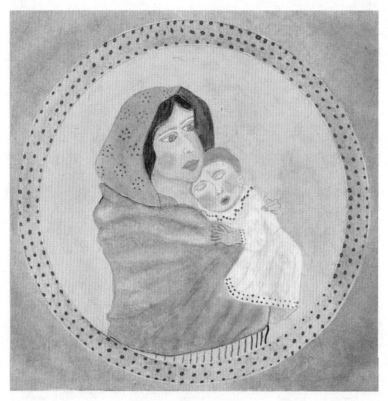

These sacred women, the *qadishtu,* whose behavior according to their own ancestral beliefs was of a noble and sacred nature, have been described as "ritual prostitutes" in most historical descriptions, not only negating the sanctity of their role and position, but warping the cultural and religious expression of an entire people. The Old Testament refers to these sacred women as harlots and adulteresses; their ancient customs are described as whoring.

Yet the women of Israel continued to follow these ancient and deeply ingrained religious practices, despite the condemnation and threats of the Hebrew leaders.

They continued to serve the Goddess in the same ancient ways throughout the biblical times and long after the Hebrews' settled in the land of Judah. In fact, the customs, rites and ceremonies of the Goddess religion remained an aspect of the religious worship at the temple in Jerusalem, the temple that had been built by the Hebrews and claimed for Yahweh alone.

For thousands of years it had been natural among Mediterranean, Near and Middle Eastern people that female kinship and custom was the order of the day…and perhaps because of this, there was an inherent lack of concern with the paternity of children.

In response, the Levite priests, who had great contempt for any woman who was neither married nor virgin, devised the concept of sexual morality. Premarital virginity was demanded for women under penalty of death. Marital fidelity for women was also demanded under penalty of death. The Levites wanted total control over the knowledge of paternity of children.

All women were therefore publicly designated as the private property of either their father or husband. Any woman who did not abide by these new laws of morality, or did not profess allegiance to Yahweh, was labeled a harlot or adulteress, which eventually became the ultimate sin.

This all encompassing social restructuring was nothing more than a bold political maneuver staged over time to access and gain power over land and property. Without virginity before marriage and stringent sexual restraints afterward, male possession of name and assets as well as divine right to the throne could not exist.

Merlin Stone's book *When God was a Woman* registers a long list of rules established between 1,000 and 600 B.C. stipulating severe punishments for Hebrew women who deviate from the law, including shameful and excruciating death.

Women who cannot prove virginity before marriage are to be stoned to death by all the men in the city. A Levite daughter was to be burned. Men could marry as many as they wished at any time, but women who commit adultery were put to death with their lover.

The rape of a virgin was honored as a declaration of ownership and brought about a forced marriage. The victim of rape, if married or betrothed, was killed with her attacker. A man could divorce his wife for any reason at any time.

In contrast, among the Goddess cultures, if a man took a second woman after his first wife had given birth, he was put out of the house without any possessions...

Once the economic and social sovereignty of women was undermined, they were forced by the new male kinship into being reliant on one constant partner or provider who "ruled over her" and to whom she dutifully and obediently submitted.

"SHE WHO HOLDS THE REINS OF KINGS, WHO GIVES THE SCEPTER, THE THRONE, THE YEAR OF REIGN TO ALL KINGS..."

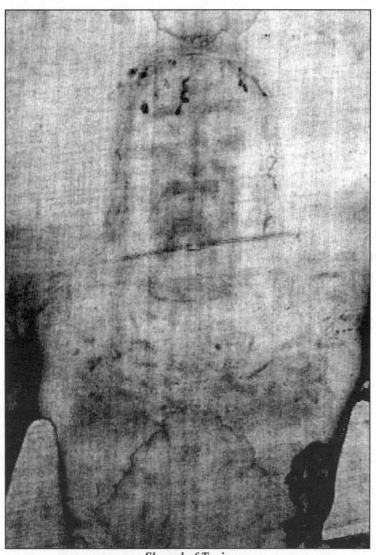
Shroud of Turin

One of the most ancient and universal practices recorded among the diverse peoples who revered the Goddess is the ritual of the dying son or consort. This ritual drama was enacted yearly and centered on the sacrifice of a king, consort or son of the High Priestess, who was then left alone to grieve.

Though the names and scenes vary, the essential theme remains the same. Quite simply, the High Priestess chose a new consort in the spring of each year. The *hieros gamos*, or sacred marriage, was enacted. This annual ceremonial drama included both oral, and later written dialogue for each of the roles. After their sexual union the young man assumed the role of king. He is given the title "Shepherd of the Land," and the Goddess fashions for him a good destiny. His life now entails the joys of "spending long days in her sacred lap."

This son/lover/king as shepherd appears over and over again in various versions throughout time. The king was killed, died or was banished, and the High Priestess was left alone in her sorrow. His resurrection was celebrated the following spring. Sometimes the story entails a mother and daughter, as in the myth of Demeter and Persepina.

Isis/Osiris - Innana/Dumuzi - Ishtar/Tammuz

Cybele/Attis - Demeter/Persepina

Later, instead of dying, the king/consort was humiliated in the temple, stripped of his garments, and beaten in the face. Good fortune was predicted for the year ahead if tears came to his eyes while being struck. The king's tears and his sweat and blood were believed to be necessary and magical substances that brought fertility and abundance to the earth. This mythic poetic ritual drama, or divine pattern, goes back to remote antiquity and represents the theological ideas developed and annually re-enacted by ancient peoples who were in intimate connection with the seasonal changes of the earth and sky. The ritual sacrifice of an annual king is found in the most ancient legends of Sumer and Egypt, and continued to exist in the Near East until the early centuries of Christianity. These ancient myths grew out of the *"collective psyche of our ancestors and are relevant to our own psyches today." Charlene Spretnak.*

Merlin Stone and others have speculated that these ancient myths may have evolved in the present time as the annual mourning for the passion and death of Jesus.

In our village we pace the 14 Stations of the Cross each Friday during Lent. We walk along with Jesus and Mary as they tread the road to Calvary. Jesus is stripped of his garments and crowned with thorns. He is mocked and beaten and made to carry a heavy cross. He falls repeatedly under its weight. He meets his women followers and consoles them. The blood on his face is wiped by Veronica. He comes upon his mother and bears the anguish and misery in her eyes. He is nailed to the cross and dies between two thieves. Finally he is taken down from the cross and placed in a tomb.

We experience his agony and humiliation. We share the sorrow and heartache of his mother. We sing an ancient chant in a minor key. Most of us shed tears. Some of us cry openly. On Easter morning there will be a great celebration. Christ is risen from the dead! All of life has been renewed!

That this enactment of ritual drama may be an evolution of much more ancient myths in no way detracts from the depth of its meaning. Nor does it diminish the historical Jesus and Mary or their divine message of love and redemption. It merely points out that as Christianity developed, myths and sacred stories about Jesus' life and death may have taken on symbolic significance that resonated with the people of the ancient world; and that these primordial stories are still resonating in the hearts and minds of people today.

The High Priestess of the temple held exceptional political power and position. Among the people she was the Goddess. The king held his position because he was married to, or was the son of, the sacred Priestess or the Goddess. Following the military conquests of these lands, the invaders married the high priestesses to acquire legitimacy and the power of the throne in the eyes of the people.

Among King Solomon's 700 recorded legal wives were many princesses from other lands. Thus he acquired the title and right to rule their territories. Marrying into wealth and power is one way of getting hold of it, and the Indo-Europeans used this strategy well. As time went on and the invaders infiltrated, the Priestesses of the Goddess lost a long list of their former privileges.

In the story of Gilgamesh, written about 2,500 B.C., we are told how he spurns the high priestess, lists all her past lovers and the dismal fate they met, and then insults the Goddess. He wants to be king for a more extended time. One year will not suffice. He wants immortality. This ancient story is an account of the ongoing confrontation between two cultures waged over many centuries.

The classic Greek myths were built upon older, more ancient Goddess-centered myths. The earlier names of the reigning Goddesses remained the same, but their attributes were grossly distorted. They were "married to" or otherwise subdued or disempowered by the new male gods introduced by the Indo-Europeans. The Greek myths tell the story of the subjugation of the female, and her ways of worship, in favor of the new male-oriented system of government and religion.

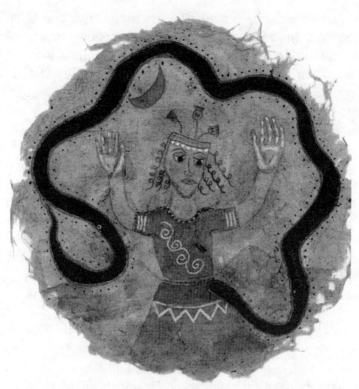

"DIVINE SERPENT LADY"
"GREAT MOTHER SERPENT OF HEAVEN"

As we have seen, the ancient Goddess religion developed over many thousands of years and was exceedingly rich in intricate symbolism.

Serpents, sacred boughs or fruit trees and women who prophesied or took advice from serpents were all images that conveyed the presence of the Goddess. These images were well known symbols of the female deity since the most ancient of days. Many other images conveyed her presence as well, such as the phases of the moon, stars and sun, swirling and coiling designs, chevrons and meandering lines, water fowl of all kinds, the dove, and many trees, plants, animals and landscapes.

The snake associated with a female in the Near and Middle East was linked to wisdom and prophetic counsel. An ancient shrine to the Serpent Lady on the Sinai Peninsula contains a prayer to her written in both Egyptian and Semitic script. Her worship was widespread. One of the earliest forms of Inanna, known as Nina, was that of a serpent goddess in the most ancient Sumerian period.

This same Serpent Lady may have been used to placate the Hebrew people during their travail in the desert. During one particular trial, when many of the people were dying after having been bitten by snakes which had descended on them in great multitudes, Moses was told by Yahweh to create a bronze serpent and to hang it from a stick. We are told in the Bible that this serpent had healing powers and was used to heal the people and to prevent their deaths.

After the Hebrews settled in Canaan and built their temple, they placed the serpent Moses had made in a sacred place within it. This "brazen serpent" was still in the temple at Jerusalem 700 years later when Hezekiah finally destroyed it as a "pagan abomination."

The serpent was clearly a symbol of and strongly identified with the Goddess religion, and it had been kept in the holy temple of Jerusalem, central place of worship for the Hebrews, for more than 700 years after their arrival in the Promised Land. This is the same temple where in 600 B.C. there were vessels for Ashoreth and Baal, the asherah, and the women weeping for Tammuz. Clearly the two religions were coexisting side by side through all these centuries, and under the very same sacred roof.

Even at the time of Christ we find the elder Prophetess, Anna, residing at the temple when the infant Jesus was presented for his initial blessings, according to the Jewish law. Elderly women not only held prophetic and advisory positions but they were associated with both mental and physical healing. It was Innana, after all, who gave the precious gift of *"eldership"* to civilization.

Marija Gimbutus beautifully explains in *The Language of the Goddess* that the spiraling, coiling snake represents life force, it is a seminal symbol, epitome of the worship of life on this earth. It is not the body of the snake that is sacred, but the energy it exudes. This same energy is found in spirals, swirls, vines, growing trees, phalluses and stalagmites but is especially concentrated in the snake, and so it is the most potent symbol of this life energy that permeates all things.

The snake is something primordial and mysterious coming out of the depths of the waters where life begins. Its seasonal renewal, shedding its old skin and hibernating, make it a symbol of the continuity of life. Chevrons, x's, aquatic symbols, zigzags, meanders, and streams accompany snakes and the Snake Goddess according to the *Language of the Goddess.*

According to Gimbutas, there is an intimate connection between the ancient Bird Goddess and Snake Goddess. They share similar symbols that have lasted until historic times. In ancient Greece, Athena's attributes were birds and snakes. Goddess of Wisdom, Athena is often depicted with a serpent peering out from behind her shield or by her side.

Athena, Brave One, Wise One
Warrior Goddess, Mother of Courage,
One with Gaia, guardian of the oracles of prophecy.
Ancient weaver and craftswoman, you invented the pottery wheel, tamed the wild horse, and taught the arts of medicine and healing.
Woman alone who takes no husband, complete of herself.

The Erechtheum, considered home of Athena's snake, was a special building beside her temple, the Parthenon.

Hera, also said to have descended from the Snake Goddess, was called *"origin of all things."* Her name is cognate with Hora, which means *"season."* Hera's sanctuaries were erected in valleys at the estuaries to rivers or near the sea and were surrounded by pastures. Paestum, a magnificently preserved ancient temple grounds on the western coast of Italy, is exactly such a place.

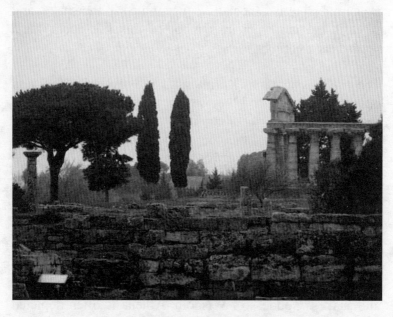

Hera, honored as Holy Heifer.
Founder of Civilization
Goddess of Battle
You wear a crown of marjoram on your head
and give the gifts of sacred healing plants.
You assign our lifelong mate and make our union strong.
You were a Great Mother long before you married Zeus.

Offerings to Hera include terracotta snakes, horned animals and calves. Homer called her "cow faced." Hera appears crowned and possesses magical healing plants. Through the touch of a plant she can restore life. Egyptian Hathor was depicted as a cow and was also described as the primeval serpent who ruled the world... Shrines dedicated to these two Goddesses often stand together.

Fertility and regeneration, healing and creating life anew are all aspects of the snake. When depicted as winding upward the snake symbolized increase, ascending life force, the tree of life and the spinal cord and was a potent symbol of healing.

A staff with a snake wrapped around it, as in Hermes magical healing cane, or *kerykeion*, or the staff held by Asklepios, in whose name temples for dreaming and healing were erected in ancient Greece and Italy, or Moses' bronze serpent wrapped on the stick in the desert, all symbolized and possessed this healing and regenerating power. Babylonian Ishtar, the Prophetess, sits on a throne holding a staff with two snakes coiled around it.

Representations of snakes in the form of round stamp seals with snake motifs have been known since the Upper Paleolithic and continue to be seen through the Neolithic. As early as 7,000 B.C., there were shrines to the Snake Goddess, and the coil served as the insignia of the Goddess in her epiphany as a snake. Since this antiquity the crown, symbol of wealth and wisdom, is the most consistent feature seen in representations of the Snake Goddess.

Paintings on the walls of a cave in Porto Badisco in Apulia, Italy depict mystifying creatures painted in black with limbs ending in snake spirals. Many small statuettes were recovered from the Palace at Knossos. These female figurines have their gowns and aprons adorned with spirals and snakes are crawling over their arms. Snakes wrap around their waist or abdomen and peer from atop their headdresses.

The primeval image of the snake is also seen in the ancient art of the Celtic peoples, in ancient Greek and Minoan art, and in Scotland, Germany, throughout Scandinavia and among indigenous North American peoples.

A snake living in or under the house means happiness and prosperity for all who live within. The snake was considered the guardian of the home, it was clairvoyant, therefore knew the futures of all the members in the family. The snake also brought connection to the ancestors and symbolized the continuation of life between the generations. Because it shed its skin, its teachings were that of immortality as seen in the natural cycles of nature. Its presence ensures the fertility of the family, farm and animals, and some people even kept one under their marriage bed.

Among the ancient peoples, the Snake Goddess was the oracular deity who interpreted dreams of the future. Ancient Babylonian myths recount the tale of Tiamat, described as a serpent, who possessed the tablets of destiny.

Tiamat
Ancient Mesopotamian Goddess
revered as Mother of Mothers
Known also as Nammu, Asherah, Atagaris and Nuneit.
Possessor of the tablets of destiny
Much later murdered by Murduk
who arrogantly pierced her with his evil winds
and then pretended that he made the world.

Among the Egyptians the association of snake and Goddess is so ancient that the hieroglyphic sign for Goddess was a cobra. She was known as the eye of insight and wisdom.

From the earliest times the sacred Goddess at the shrine in Delphi supplied divine revelation as spoken by the priestess, or Sybil, who served her. One means of divination was incubation. The priestess slept in the holy shrine with her ear to the ground, listening to the murmurs of the earth. This priestess spoke in rhythmic oracles of divine wisdom. Coiled around the tripod stool upon which she sat while making her pronouncements was a snake, known as Python. The city of Delphi was known as Pytho in even earlier times.

Archaeological evidence shows that the earliest temple at Delphi had been built by women, and it was recorded that at this most sacred shrine the Goddess was revered as Gaia, Primeval Prophetess. This holy site of divination, and others identified with the Goddess for eons, were later confiscated by priests of Zeus and Apollo, both of whom are described in their myths as having killed the serpent of the Goddess Gaia, *Oldest of the Holy Ones*.

Gaia, Primeval Prophetess,
Ancient Earth
Universal Mother who created heaven, earth and sea

The many sculptures and reliefs of women fighting against men (the women are usually called Amazons) found at this shrine are thought to depict the early battles between the Goddess worshipers and the invading Indo-Europeans. These are our soul sisters of long ago defending the Goddess with all their apparently considerable might.

Merlin Stone recounts the work of William Hoast of Florida in *When God Was a Woman*. The Serpentarian has spent his life working with and studying snakes and was quoted in Life Magazine as saying that poisonous snake venom has a chemical makeup similar to mescaline, psilocybin and LSD. After being bitten he reports, "I find myself making up wonderful verses – my mind has extraordinary powers." It is interesting to note that the oracles given by the priestesses of the ancient sacred shrines were also offered in rhyming verse.

A venomous snake bite usually leads to swelling, paralysis, breathing difficulty and may even result in death. But, according to Hoast, if immunized first, and then bitten by a cobra or other elapid, one experiences an emotional and mental state like that brought on by hallucinogenic drugs. It seems that the bite of a certain sacred snake can offer gifts of insight into the inner workings of the universe.

Our sister priestesses of many centuries ago were trained to listen to the quiet whisper of a revered snake, to hear the murmurs of the living earth or to breath in sacred vapors oozing from a crevice in the floor, and by these methods, and others, peer into the future. They offered advice based on their direct communication with the Deity who possessed the wisdom of the universe. This deity was the Snake Goddess.

The wise counsel offered by the priestess in the form of divine revelation was an aspect of the Goddess religion since the most ancient times. The snake had been the symbol of this divine revelation and prophesy since remote antiquity.

And Yahweh told the serpent "I will put enmity between you and the woman, and between your seed and her seed."

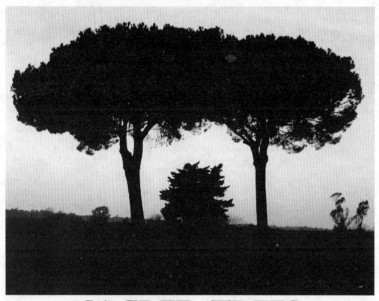

SACRED TREES

Considered a manifestation of divine presence since remote antiquity, trees have long been an object of veneration as well as a symbol of the communication between the heavenly, earthly and lower realms. A verdant tree branch or bough represents regeneration, rebirth and protection in ancient stories from many varied cultures.

In some of the oldest stories the fig tree was known as the living body of Hathor on earth. It was said that to eat the fruit of this tree was to eat the flesh and blood of the Goddess, among whose titles was *Lady of the Sycamore.*

Eating of the tree of the Goddess, which stood by each altar (a branch was passed around in the temple and its fruit eaten as a form of communion), was as dangerously "pagan" as were her sexual customs and prophetic serpents.

Ancient Minoan and Mycenaean stone seals and rings show many images of the priestesses of the Goddess tending to fruit tress, as if in blessed devotion.

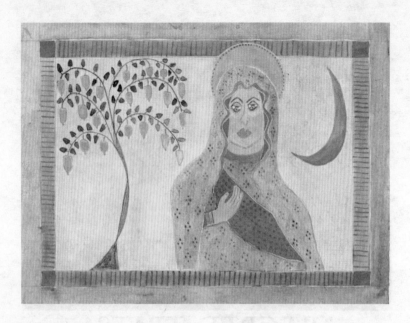

Stories from classical Greece tell us of Hera and her fruit tree with the serpent Ladon coiled around it. This tree we are told was given to Hera by Gaia, Primeval Prophetess.

Among the ancient grape-cultivating Italic tribes, the elm tree was sacred. *Ulmus* was used to support young grape vines as they grew, and this tree eventually became the *alma mater* of the Wine-god, Dionysius. Among the early Mediterranean peoples, the apple was considered the sacred fruit of Venus, Goddess of Love.

> *Aphrodite,*
> *White Bird of Heaven*
> *essence of erotic love*
> *Sacred Star who wears a wreath of*
> *poppies and myrtle leaves*
> *You are the love of motherhood*
> *and the oldest of fates*

Ancient people honored not only the light aspects of the Goddess, but they honored the dark as well.

The willow was the sacred tree of Hecate, Circe, Hera and Persephone, all of whom represented the Death aspect of the Triple Goddess.

> *Hecate, dark side of the moon*
> *Queen of the Dead, Oldest of Old*
> *The mighty energies of a million hearts*
> *are contained within you.*
> *Holy Enchantress*
> *Guide of Transformations*
> *You give power to the spoken word*
> *You are a sorcerer and witch.*

In India this dark aspect of the Goddess is known as Kali.

> *She is Black as Night*
> *called Sleep, called Dream*
> *Joyous Dancer Among the Dead*
> *Fierce Warrior Woman*
> *One Who Dispels Fear*
> *Great Mother Time*
> *She wears a garland of heads around her neck*
> *a belt of hands around her waist*
> *there is blood upon her lips*
> *She is a mother born of anger and at world's end it will be*
> *Kali gathering the seeds for a new creation.*

These dark Goddesses were all interchangeable with the Moon Goddess, known by the Romans as Minerva, and to whom the willow was also sacred.

In *The White Goddess*, a historical grammar of poetic myth, Robert Graves says that the palm tree was the Tree of Life in the Babylonian Garden of Eden story. "*Its Hebrew name is 'Tamar' – Tamar was the Hebrew equivalent of Great Goddess, Istar or Ashtaroth; and the Arabians adored the palm of Nejran as a goddess, annually draping it in women's clothes and ornaments.*"

In the Bible we learn that the Lord grew every species of plant in the Garden of Eden, including the Tree of Life and the Tree of Knowledge of Good and Evil, which stood in the heart of the garden. The first humans, Adam and Eve, are placed in the garden and told not to eat the fruit of the Tree of Knowledge of Good and Evil. This was understood by the people to mean the sacred tree, the asherah, the fruits of which were communally eaten as a form of "communion."

"So into the myth of how the world began, the story that the Levites offered as the explanation of the creation of all existence, they place the advisory serpent and the woman who accepted its counsel, eating of the tree that gave her the understanding of what "only the gods knew" - the secret of sex, and how to create life. Yahweh's followers destroyed her temples and shrines wherever they could, murdered who they could not convert and the Levite priests wrote the creation tale." Merlin Stone

It is always the conquerors' version of history that we hear.

It was made clear by the Hebrew priests that the woman ate the fruit upon advice from the serpent, which until now has been understood as the instrument of divine counsel. They wanted the snake to be perceived as a source of evil. The oracular priestesses, the prophetess identified with the sacred serpent for millennia, we're now told have caused the downfall of the entire human race.

"The new, patriarchal religion co-opted the older mythic symbols and inverted their meaning: The female, Eve, was now weak-willed and treacherous; the sacred bough was now forbidden; and the serpent, symbol of regeneration and renewal with its shedding skins, was now the embodiment of evil." Charlene Spretnak

Woman, once advisor, guide, mentor, wise counselor, and human interpreter of divine will, is now to be feared, hated, doubted or ignored. According to Judaic and Christian theology, a woman's judgment led to disaster for all.

The new myths said that male ownership and control of submissive and obedient women was to be regarded as the natural state of the human species. They asserted that male supremacy was divinely ordained since the beginning of existence. Dominion over women, and indeed all the earth, was the first proclamation of this new male creator.

According to these new stories, women were assigned the role of sexual temptress. *"Cunning, conniving, arouser of physical desire in men, she who offers an appealing, but dangerous fruit."* Merlin Stone

Sex became immoral. Judaism, and later Christianity, developed theological ideas that promoted guilt about being a human being with sexual needs. Our innate human sexuality, formerly celebrated as sacred, was no longer considered a natural biological desire that encouraged the reproduction of the species but was viewed as "women's fault" by the new male religion, which regarded procreation as shameful or sinful.

Proof of our guilt was made evident by the natural pain of childbirth, which came to be seen as a curse and our eternal chastisement. *"In pain you shall bring forth children, yet your desire shall be for your husband and he shall rule over you."* Genesis

The myth of Eve pierces the wild hearts of woman. It hurts our feelings, our minds, our bodies and our spirits. The myth of Eve portrays women as spiritually weak and mentally impoverished.

The laws and attitudes originally designed to eradicate the Goddess religions, female sexual autonomy and matrilineal descent, are still present in the structure of contemporary religion and government today. According to Jews, Christians and Muslims, man is master by divine right, not only over women, but all of creation.

"By law, public sentiment and religion from the time of Moses down to the present day, woman has never been thought of as other than a piece of property to be disposed of at the will of man." Susan B. Anthony, 1860

When we become aware of the earlier female-oriented religious expressions of people that far pre-dated the Old Testament Creation and Adam and Eve myths, our eyes, and our wild hearts, begin to open. And with this opening our deep personal and collective wound begins to heal. This healing can clear away centuries of accumulated confusion and misunderstanding.

Our general education system and popular literature do not reflect the existence, or importance, of these earlier cultures, perhaps because knowledge of them seems to refute what we conceive of as the *"natural, divinely ordained role of women."* Despite the reason for this centuries old censorship, thanks to the work of the scholars whose words are liberally strewn throughout these pages, and many others, this knowledge is now "out of the bag" and into the open. It is flowing into mainstream culture like streams into a river when the snows are melting in spring.

Together we are giving birth to a new era, a new consciousness. We are a part of bringing it forth onto the planet and into the minds and hearts of the people.

The Feminine face of God is shining from our faces. She is calling from our wild hearts. Her voice is our voice and we will not be silenced. Her presence cannot be obliterated. She is as present today as she ever was. She is pregnant with the power of waiting. And she can wait no longer. She is giving birth to us and we are giving birth to her.

Lift up your voices in joy and gladness. Lift them up in thanksgiving and healing. Hear them lilting across the eons of life on this planet.

Make the joyful sounds of birthing peace for all creation...

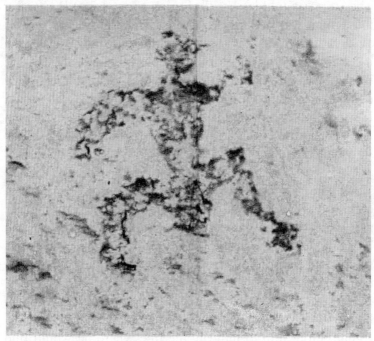

Petroglyph of a woman giving birth, Indian Rock, *Solon, Maine*

THE CUMAEAN SYBIL

SHE WHO SPEAKS TO THE SOULS OF THE DEAD

Virgil's epic poem, *The Aeneid,* written between 29-19 B.C. recounts a story that was an ancient tale even then, regarding the heroic Trojan prince Aeneas, whose mother was the Goddess Venus. The revered and respected Cumaean Sybil, sacred priestess and prophetess, plays an important role in this classic myth, which contains many elements from much earlier days…

The story, as told by Virgil, begins about 1,200 B.C., after the Trojan war had ended. Aeneas fled Troy carrying his aged father on his back and leading his young son by the hand as his wife Creusa followed close behind, though she was soon lost. Along with a band of Trojan soldiers, they escaped to safety on Mount Ida. In the forests of Mount Ida they built ships and set forth in search of a new home. After many travels and travails, Aeneas landed at a place in Italy called Cumae. There dwelt the Sibyl.

Now, the Sibyls were extraordinary virgin priestesses endowed with profound wisdom and the gift of prophecy; and when Aeneas consulted the Cumaean Sybil, she told him that he must visit the Underworld of Pluto to learn his future fate. But before leaving he was to gather a golden bough, which he was to carry in his hand to keep him safe. Aeneas searched in the forest long and hard for the golden bough until two doves, his mother's sacred birds, came flying before him to indicate the tree where he would find the shining branch. Guarded with the protective bough and guided by the Sybil, Aeneas passed through a dark and dismal cave, where he came to the river Styx. The Sybil convinced the ferryman to take Aeneas across, and as he did his boat groaned under the weight of a living human being. On the other side of the river stood Cerberus, the ferocious three-headed dog who was the guardian of the Underworld. The Sybil threw him a cake of honey and poppy seeds and he fell asleep, allowing for safe passage. Aeneas continued on until he came to groves of myrtle, a plant sacred to Venus, where he found all those who had ever died for love. He persisted on to the Elysian Fields where he found the spirit of his father, Anchises, and there he was allowed to see the souls of all their descendants, as yet unborn. Thus Aeneas knew he would succeed on his journey to find a new homeland.

Aeneas and his descendants reigned for fifteen generations. The last of these was Amulius, who took the throne from his brother Numitor. The grandsons of Numitor were Romulus and Remus, the mythological founders of Rome...

Cumae is an antediluvian settlement located just above the stunning Bay of Poluzzi, on the rim of especially translucent waters about twenty miles west of Naples and a mere two hour drive from our mountain village. It was founded by the Chalchidians around 800 B.C., long before the rise of Rome, and is surrounded by an especially rich and fertile volcanic plain. The stunning beauty of the area inspired the early inhabitants to identify it as the mythological Elysian Fields and to designate the nearby lake, Lago d'Averno, as the entrance to the Underworld. This is the site of the celebrated Solfatara, a prehistoric and long dormant volcanic crater near Mt. Vesuvius where thermal springs and small volcanoes of hot mud still bubble up from the earth as they did in ancient times.

"The volcanic region near Vesuvius, where the whole country is cleft with chasms from which sulphurous flames arise, while the ground is shaken with pent-up vapors, and mysterious sounds issue from the bowels of the earth..."
Campania, Ancient Sites, Museo d/Napoli

This is the home of the most famous of all the Sybils, *The Sibyl of Cumae,* sometimes called by the names Amalthaea, Heraphile or Demophile. The word sibyl comes to us via Latin, from the Greek *sibylla*, meaning prophetess.

The Sybil of Cumae prophesied by "singing the fates" and then wrote her predictions down on oak leaves which were placed around the many entrances to her cave and read by anyone who wished. If the wind blew and scattered the leaves they would not be rearranged to form the original prophesy again. This is how Virgil described it:

> Arrived at Cumae, when you view the flood
> Of black Avernus, and the sounding wood,
> The mad prophetic Sibyl you shall find,
> Dark in a cave and on a rock reclined
> She sings the fates, and, in her frantic fits,
> The notes and names, inscribed, to leafs commits
> What she commits to leaf in order laid
> Before the cavern's entrance are displayed
> Unmoved they lie; but, if a blast of wind
> Without, or vapors issue from behind,
> The leafs are borne aloft in liquid air,
> And she resumes no more her museful care,
> Nor gathers from the rocks her scattered verse,
> Nor sets in order what the winds disperse.
> Thus, many not succeeding, most upbraid
> The madness of the visionary maid,
> And with loud curses leave the mystic shade.

As we've seen, long ago wise women inhabited shrines, temples and caves, and were blessed with the gift of prophecy. They read the signs of nature and were able to portend the future. The Sibyl in Cumae was especially revered, because she was able not only to prophesize and advise but to communicate with the souls of the dead and to guide others to do so. Although our knowledge of these sacred women is somewhat obscured by time, many myths exist about them that give us some clues. In the sixth century B.C., Heraclitus recorded: *The Sibyl, with frenzied mouth uttering things not to be laughed at, unadorned and unperfumed, yet reaches to a thousand years with her voice.*

The renowned Cumaean Sibyl is written about in the works of Virgil, *The Eclogues* as well as the *Aeneid*, in Ovid's *Metamorphoses* and Petronius' *The Satyricon*. She was featured in paintings by Michelangelo, Van Eck and many other artists, and her image adorns altar pieces, illuminated manuscripts and even the ceiling of the Sistine Chapel, where she is prominently displayed among the Old Testament prophets.

Venerated by pagans and Christians alike, the Cumaean Sybil is believed to have prophesied, among many other things, the birth of Jesus. Constantine, the Christian emperor, interpreted the whole of Virgil's *The Eclogues* as a reference to the coming of Christ and, in his first address to the assembly, quoted a long passage of the Sibylline Book (*Book 8*) containing an acrostic in which the initials from a series of verses read: Jesus Christ Son of God Savior, Cross.

The Cumaean Sibyl we are told, inhabited a cave with one hundred mouths. This ancient *Cave of the Sibyl* was lost, or perhaps hidden, for more than two thousand years, but was found and excavated in 1932. It is now accessible by a passage found within the ruins of the original Cumaean settlement. Her sacred grotto, a trapezoidal passage over 131 meters long, runs parallel to the side of a hill and was cut out of the volcanic stone by hand, using simple tools. The early stories tell us that she lived for one thousand years, and some say the Cumaean Sybil can still be heard within her sanctuary today. Indeed, the Sybil herself prophesied that her voice as well as her sayings would remain there throughout the ages.

Ovid recounts the story in *Metamorphoses*: As Aeneas and the Sibyl came back up to earth after their adventure in the Underworld he said to her: "Whether thou be a goddess or a mortal beloved by the gods, by me thou shalt always be held in reverence. When I reach the upper air, I will cause a temple to be built to thy honor, and will myself bring offerings."

"I am no goddess," said the Sibyl; "I have no claim to sacrifice or offering. I am mortal; yet if I had accepted the love of Apollo, I might have been immortal. He promised me the fulfillment of my wish, if only I would consent to be his. I took a handful of sand, and holding it forth, said, 'Grant me to see as many birthdays as there are sand-grains in my hand.'

"Unfortunately I did not ask for enduring youth. This also he would have granted, if I accepted his love, but offended at my refusal, he allowed me to grow old. My youth and youthful strength fled long ago. I have lived seven hundred years, and to equal the number of sand-grains in my hand, I have still to see three hundred springs and three hundred harvests. My body shrinks up as the years increase, and in time, I shall be lost to sight, but my voice will remain, and future ages will respect my sayings."

The Cumaen Sybil tells us that she resisted uniting with the Greek god Apollo, and instead stood her ground. She is firmly and wholly of the Old World.

Another tale recounts how the Sybil of Cumae walked to Rome to sell nine books of her prophesies to the King of the Tarquins. The following version is a summary of the tale as told by Amy Friedman:

For many years, beneath the temple of Jupiter in Rome, the Sibylline books were protected in a closely guarded vault. These books contained great wisdom and predictions of what the future held for their land and people. The Sibylline books, the priests said, were precious beyond any treasure and were consulted during times of natural disaster and when hardships came.

The Cumaean Sibyl had an open and wild heart. She was wild-eyed, wild-haired and wild-tongued. One day, she came to see the king, Tarquin the Elder. She had nine books to sell. "In these nine books," she said, "is contained the destiny of Rome."

Tarquin the Elder laughed at the old woman. He did not believe she could predict the future, nor that these books contained the destiny of the world. Nevertheless he asked, "How much money do you want for your books?" "Nine bags of gold," she answered. The king and his advisers roared with laughter.

"The future of your world lies within them," she repeated, but seeing that he did not wish to buy her books, she started a fire, and into this fire she hurled three of her books. She then turned away and walked the many days journey back to her grotto in Cumae.

It was another year before the Sibyl returned offering six books for sale. "Six books that contain the rest of the destiny of Rome."

"How much?" the king asked her. "Nine bags of gold," she said. "Too much," Tarquin answered, and so, once again, she built a fire and threw into it three more books. Then she walked away, crossing the wide open lands that lay between Rome and Cumae.

The next year, she returned to see the king once again. This time she brought with her the three remaining books. "Three books remain," she said, "and I will sell these to you for nine bags of gold."

Now the king's advisers gathered around consulting among themselves. They were worried that the Sibyl would burn the very last of her predictions. What if what she said were true? What if they might know their future? What if they were throwing away their opportunity to read their destinies as well as the destiny of Rome?

"You must buy the books," the advisers told their king, and so he did, paying the old Sibyl nine bags of gold. When the king and his advisers read the three books that remained, they realized that this wild old woman was truly a great Sibyl, prophetess of the future. The king sent at once for her and had her returned to his court. "Please," Tarquin begged her, "will you rewrite the other six books?"

"No," she said. "You have chosen your destiny, and I cannot change that."

The three remaining books of the Cumaean Sybil were lost when the Temple of Jupiter burned in 80 B.C. Sibylline prophecies from all parts of Italy and Greece were subsequently sought to replace them. These were saved in the rebuilt temple and eventually moved to the Temple of Apollo on the Palatine Hill, where they remained and were carefully consulted throughout the Imperial Period.

The books were purposely burned in 405 A.D. by the General Flavius Stilicho, who regarded them as pagan and therefore evil. When the Visigoths sacked Rome five years later many Romans lamented the loss of the Sybil's prophesies, claiming that the invasion of the city was evidence of the wrath of the gods.

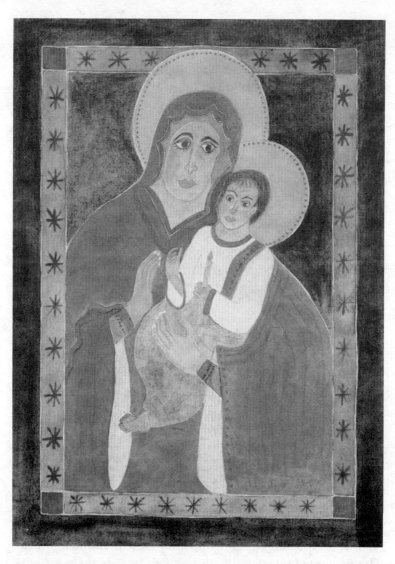

For unto us a child is born, a son is given; and the government shall be upon his shoulder, and his name shall be called...the mighty God, the Prince of Peace. Isaiah, 9:6

THE PRINCE OF PEACE

Jesus was born into an era of great political unrest and uncertainty. Because of the turmoil of the times, the Jews longed for the savior who had been promised them by Isaiah, a promise repeated in the Book of Daniel and again in the Book of Enoch. This *Messiah*, they hoped, would rectify all their present ills and oppressions under Roman rule.

A charismatic faith healer named Jesus of Nazareth began teaching around the shores of Galilee and in the villages nearby. His message was a message of love and forgiveness. He spoke simply, beautifully and poetically. He was especially compassionate to those most in need. And he healed the sick and infirm among them. These qualities endeared him to the local people, and he soon gained a following.

And he came down with them, and stood in the plain, and the company of his disciples and a great multitude of people out of all Judea and Jerusalem, and from the sea coast of Tyre and Sidon, which came to hear him, and to be healed of their diseases...and they were healed.
Luke 6:17-18

The disenfranchised found that Jesus valued their worth as much or more than the richest among them. The sick flocked to him for healing.

Women especially found that they had a friend in Jesus. His teachings resonated with women; he saw them as equal in every way and counted many women among his friends, followers and disciples. Jesus treated women with kindness and respect, no matter what their social status.

"When thou wert in the world, Lord, thou didst not despise women, but didst always help them and show them great compassion." Theresa of Avila

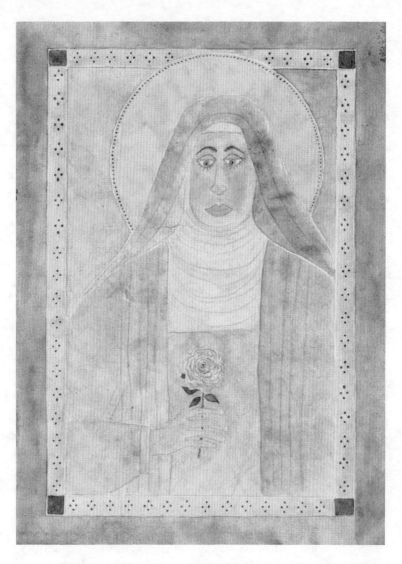

His teachings on marriage declare it to be a lifelong bond of faithfulness between two people. When Jesus said, *"What therefore God hath joined together, let no man rent asunder." Mathew 19:6,* his words were meant to protect women, who were without protection by the laws of the time. Men could divorce a wife for something as trivial as not cooking a tasteful meal, exchange an aging wife for a younger one or rid themselves of a woman unable to conceive.

"Judge not, and ye shall not be judged...forgive and ye shall be forgiven." Luke 6: 37

Jesus preached nonviolence, forgiveness and unconditional love, and he instructed his disciples to *contemplate*. His teachings emphasized mercy, empathy and compassion. He promised his followers entry into the coming Kingdom of God.

When asked by a Pharisee which of the 613 laws of Leviticus he thought most important, Jesus answered, *"Thou shalt love the Lord thy God with all thy heart and with all thy soul and with all thy mind. This is the first and greatest Commandment. And the second is like unto it. Thou shalt love thy neighbor as thyself. On these two Commandments hang all the law and the prophets." Matthew 22:37-40*

Jesus was a wise and gentle teacher who asked his followers to renounce their preconceived ideas. In the simple words of the people, rather than that of a priestly class, Jesus ministered to their hearts and souls. His language was rich in image, emotion and metaphor; his poetic aphorisms were easily remembered. In fact neither Jesus, nor any of his disciples, wrote anything down. Jesus instructed his followers to commit his sermons to memory, to memorize them. He asked them to believe in Him.

"I am come a light into the world, that whosoever believeth in me should not abide in darkness." John 12:46

Jesus' electrifying sermons and radical wisdom stories provoked fear and loathing among both the Jewish and

Roman authorities who eventually conspired to rid themselves of the threat they perceived he posed.

"But woe unto you who are rich, for you have received your consolation. Woe unto you who are full, for you shall hunger. Woe unto you who laugh now, for you shall mourn and weep." Luke 6: 24-25

Jesus' life, his acts, his revolutionary teachings, his compassionate healings and magnetic presence are still reverberating in the world today.

But I say to you, love your enemies, do good to them which hate you. Bless them that curse you, and pray for them that despitefully use you…And as you would have it be done to you, do ye also to them likewise." Luke 6:27-28, 31

His prayerful passion in the sacred olive garden he loved and from where he had given many sermons among the birds and trees, his blessed gift of the Eucharist at the last supper, his betrayal by a member of his own close knit circle, the cruel treatment he endured at the hands of the authorities and his crucifixion, death and resurrection became the central themes in the new stories of Christianity and changed the flow of all human culture that followed.

"The heroic end of Christ's life mirrored familiar stories of the dying and returning gods such as Osirus, Adonis, Attis, and Dumuzi. Each was accompanied in his life by the Goddess in some form: Isis with Osirus, Venus with Adonis, Cybele with Attis and Inanna with Dumuzi." Charlene Spretnak

That Jesus the man had died, and risen three days later, emerging as the Divine Christ, brought into the world a new idea of immense beauty, grace, mystery and power. It resonated in the hearts and minds of most who heard of it.

Though the ancient story line was continued, it had received an entirely fresh and unique twist. It had come in contact with Jesus and Mary.

Jesus, the Redeemer, had been a prophet, teacher and miracle worker. His mother, Mary, was his first teacher, disciple and supporter. The magnitude and meaning of their message in Western culture is indicated by the fact that our accounting of modern time begins with Mary giving birth to Jesus.

Christianity emerged from the union of the two most dominant religions at the time, which were Judaism and the Goddess religion. It did this by *"conjoining the best elements from each of the older two into a new religion. Christianity annealed seemingly incompatible opposites into one seamless creed: numinous rites and written word, mythology and history, mystery and Law."* Leonard Shlain

The teachings of Jesus reflect the relational thinking of the Goddess people. His sayings were not focused on the letter of the law, but on the feelings, longings and experiences of the heart. The words Jesus preached reveal the ultimate goal of human activity, which is eternal happiness.

*Blessed are the poor in spirit,
for theirs is the kingdom of heaven.
Blessed are they who mourn, for they shall be comforted.
Blessed are the meek, for they will inherit the earth.
Blessed are they who hunger and thirst for righteousness,
for they will be satisfied.
Blessed are the merciful, for they shall be shown mercy.
Blessed are the pure of heart, for they will see God.
Blessed are the peacemakers,
for they will be called children of God.
Blessed are they who are persecuted for righteousness'
sake, for theirs is the kingdom of heaven.*

Blessed are you when people revile you and persecute you and utter all kinds of evil against you falsely on my account. Rejoice and be glad, for your reward will be great in heaven.

Jesus was also exceedingly well versed in and obedient to the law of the Hebrew people. His roots go deep into both the rich and nourishing soil of the ancient and collective Mother line, and the prophecies, promises, written word and Law of Moses and Abraham.

Although his immediate disciples did not write down the words Jesus spoke, those who came after them did. The first writings were the Epistles, a series of apostolic letters written by Paul, formerly Saul of Tarsus. After having actively participated in the persecution of early followers of Jesus, and being present at the stoning of Stephen, one of Jesus' disciples, Saul had an epiphany. In a vision he saw the figure of Jesus and heard him ask "Saul, Saul, why are you persecuting me?" Saul changed his name to Paul and converted to Christianity.

He dedicated the rest of his life to spreading the words of Jesus, as he interpreted them. *Rejoice evermore. Pray without ceasing. In everything give thanks. 1 Thessalonians 5:16-18*

And while mainly remaining true to the message and the heart of Jesus' teachings about love, Paul did diverge. His views of women, in particular, stood in stark contrast to those that Jesus had espoused. Jesus taught equality of all. He had spoken to the Samaritan woman, rescued an adulteress who was about to be stoned, forgave the prostitute, had many women friends and supporters among his followers and disciples, was a faithful son to the end, and had a deep and meaningful relationship with Mary Magdalene.

In addition, the apostles had found solace in the company of Mary, Mother of Jesus, after his death. When the Holy Spirit descended on the disciples, they were surrounding Mary, who was acting in the role of their teacher.

Paul, however, wrote: *"Let the woman learn in silence with all subjection."* 1 Timothy 2:14

The Gospel of Mary, one of the scrolls found at the Nag Hammadi cave in Egypt, indicates that Jesus gave Mary Magdalene mystical teachings he had not shared with the others. He also authorized The Magdalene to share these teachings. Mary Magdalene not only possessed the gift of teaching, but of healing as well. Since she had been exorcised by Jesus on several occasions, and over time, she had direct knowledge of and experience with this skill. According to the Gospel of Mary, Mary Magdalene was appointed by Jesus in a vision after his resurrection to be a teacher and leader in the newly forming Christian church.

Mary Magdalene is spoken of in other scrolls found in the cave; in the Book of Thomas, the Book of Philip and in a scroll known as the Pistis Sophia. In these writings Mary Magdalene is portrayed as one of the disciples.

She is often in the role of *interpreter,* because *"she knows the scripture and the sayings of Jesus, and she discusses their meaning. In both the Pistis Sophia and the Gospel of Mary, she shares her insight and teaches the disciples. For this she is praised, but also attacked, and in some writings it is Peter who shows hostility."* Marvin Meyer, The Gospels of Mary.

Mary Magdalene's lineage appears to be that of the ancient priestesses. The unknown author of Pistis Sophia says that Mary offered her teachings *"as a woman who understood everything."*

In both the Gospel of Philip 64 and the Gospel of Mary 18, the disciples clearly state that the master loves her more than any of them. In the Gospel of Philip 59, Mary is said to be the constant companion of the master Jesus. The First Apocalypse of James 38 and 42 relates that the master had twelve male and seven female disciples.

In the first few decades after the death of Jesus, women played a prominent role in the emerging church, and in several epistles Paul himself pays homage to them. But fear that women might gain too much power in the newly forming ministry made him change his tune. His written edicts severely curtailed any authority a woman might have within the growing Christian movement. His letters, circa 40-50 A.D., exclude women from the privilege of teaching or having any authority over a congregation. He believes that women must be silent in church. He associates all women with Eve, and thus justifies his reasoning.

"For the man is not of the woman, but the woman of the man. Neither was man created for the woman, but the woman for the man." 1 Corinthians 11:9

One of the early church fathers, Origen, writing in the first century after the death of Christ and commenting on the role of women as conceived in Paul's First Letter to the Corinthians wrote, *"For it is shameful for a woman to speak in the community. Whatever she says, even if she says admirable or holy things – it comes out of the mouth of a woman." Catena of Fragments on 1 Corinthians, 74.34-37*

Paul also insisted that the church hierarchy be entirely male and had each of the male apostles and himself (he had never met Jesus) appoint a bishop. Each bishop, acting as official head of his district, would then appoint a new bishop who would eventually replace him. The bishop in

Rome, the Pope, would have authority over all of them. Thus each of the male heads of the church would be able to trace his line back to the original apostles. Though this format certainly did not resonate with the way Jesus had related to women, Paul's beliefs soon became dogma within the new religion.

"The head of every man is Christ, the head of every woman is her husband." "wives, submit to your husbands as to the Lord." Eph 5:22-24

The earliest Christians, or followers of Christ, were a diverse group of people with a broad spectrum of beliefs and practices. Their unifying mission was to become the *salt of the earth* and *the light of the world*. Among this creative and inspired diversity, two basic structures emerged: those who took the Orthodox view of Christianity, and everyone else.

Among the Gnostics, so-called to identify them as separate from the Orthodox, women had an equal role with men in conducting sacred ceremony. The Gnostics drew lots to see who would be in charge of each meeting, believing that spirit would guide the selection. These people, ascetics who lived in the desert, understood the resurrection of Christ in symbolic, and not necessarily in physical terms.

Sometime in these first centuries of Christianity, perhaps because of a rightly perceived threat, a collection of Gnostic scrolls were judiciously hidden away in an earthen jar deep inside a cave in the Egyptian desert. These scrolls, found in Nag Hammadi in the early part of the twentieth century A.D., and mentioned above, have shed a new and different light on the subject of early Christianity.

The word Gnostic means *to know*. This kind of knowing is the kind one has in one's bones. It is intuitive knowing,

knowing something thoroughly, and knowing with depth and intimacy. It is spiritual knowledge. The Gnostics depended on spirit to direct them. They called their common gatherings *Agape,* or "Love Feast," and participants exchanged the "Kiss of Peace" at the end of their services.

The Orthodox Christians lined up directly behind Paul, and all later Christian writers built upon Paul's views. They discredited the worth of women, due to Eve's supposed earlier transgression, and believed in the resurrection of Jesus in strictly literal terms. The Orthodox relied heavily on the written word and the law to guide them, adopted the Old Testament into their body of sacred works and assumed the same dominion over women and the earth as the Old Testament described.

As you might suppose, these two approaches to Christianity squared off against one another for the first couple of centuries after Christ's death, with the Orthodox unleashing an unrelenting stream of misogynistic writing and loudly denouncing the Gnostics.

Scholars commonly agree that the four Gospels, written from oral records somewhere between 60 – 110 A.D., many years after the life and death of Jesus, and also after Paul's Epistles, contain embellishments, a few later additions, as well as probable omissions and alterations due to translation, interpretation and bias of subsequent transcribers. While acknowledging that this is the case, we must also acknowledge that the Gospels contain a written record of the words and deeds of the historical teacher we know and love as our Savior and Redeemer, Jesus, Son of God, his family members, friends and associates.

"The linear thinkers favored left-brained, male-dominated patriarchies, heavy on guilt, dogma, obedience, and the

literalness of the Christ story. The intuiters were more often egalitarian and were entranced by the mythopoesis of Jesus' life and death." Leonard Shlain

In 313 A.D., the Roman Emperor Constantine decreed that Christianity would be the state religion and that the Orthodox would officially administer it. Mobs attacked Gnostic centers and destroyed their shrines and images. All Gnostic gospels were ordered burned in 367 A.D. With the Gnostics driven out, the Orthodox declared themselves the one and only true Christian Patriarchs.

"Before the lights of literacy went out in the Dark Ages, the Christian Orthodox leaders Paul, Tertullian, Jerome, and Augustine had hammered together a religion whose central themes were sin, guilt and suffering. When the lights came on again in the tenth century Europeans had leavened this with an increased respect for birth and womanhood. This revised ethos changed the character of Christianity and is best illustrated by the sharp and unexpected ascendance of Marianism, or reverence for the Blessed Mother Mary." Leonard Shlain

Although Orthodox Christianity was not about a divine female or Goddess, devotion to Mary blossomed throughout European Christendom.

Mary was defined as the Mother of God by the Council of Ephesus in 430 A.D. The Parthenon of Athens was rededicated to Mary in 600 A.D. Magnificent Gothic cathedrals and churches rose up all over Europe. In France alone, more than one hundred churches and eighty cathedrals were erected in praise of Mary, Queen of Heaven.

By the twelfth century her image led every procession and adorned homes and work places, churches and crossroads throughout western Europe.

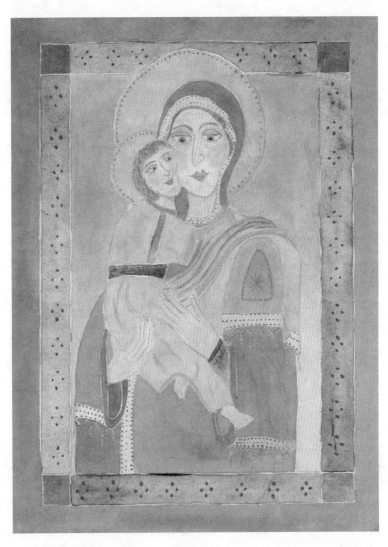

The age of chivalry was ushered in, and women, Psalters in hand, gathered together in study groups. The Inquisition was established, Popes succumbed to ridiculous excesses, and Thomas Aquinas, otherwise quite brilliant, argued that women did not possess souls. Modern, humanist thought evolved, the Protestant Reformation took place, followed by the Catholic Counter Reformation. The printing press, advances in science, the Industrial Revolution and the

Mechanical Age all altered forever the way life was lived. The Romantic poets responded by extolling love and a return to simplicity, nature and beauty. Two world wars were waged.

The atomic bomb was the pinnacle of the masculine world view, the shocking and sickening sight of its mushroom cloud a vivid warning that death for all was imminent. The photo of Earth from space made it all too clear how vulnerable we are, how precious is our planet, how dearly we want to protect it, how much we want to live.

LSD and psychedelics, meditation, Yoga and many other spiritual and practices, drawing closer to both nature and community, as well as the new quantum physics, have given us glimpses of fresh possibilities. The women's movement, environmental movement, organic agriculture, the many old and new healing modalities and the reemergence of the Goddess are all building upon these insights now.

Though dogmatic, social and political arguments will no doubt continue to rage, and loyalties severely tested, especially among church and political hierarchy, I believe the people long ago decided where their innate allegiance lay.

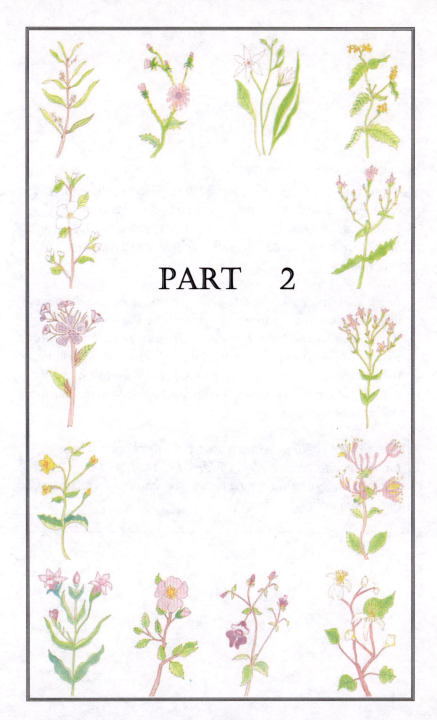

PART 2

According to the ancient stories, Jesus was a simple man, a carpenter like his step-father, Joseph. He was the son of a virgin mother, Mary, who had been presented to the temple at the age of three by her elderly parents, Ann and Joachim.

Mary was raised on the temple grounds and would have worshiped at the temple with other women, according to their ways. Although it is written into Jewish law that women are not to be within the inner sanctum of the temple, we've seen that women continued to live and worship within the temple complex throughout the centuries before and into the time of Christ.

The stories say that when it was time to choose a husband for the young temple virgin Mary, the staff held by Joseph sprouted a green leaf. Thus he was chosen from among those men being considered.

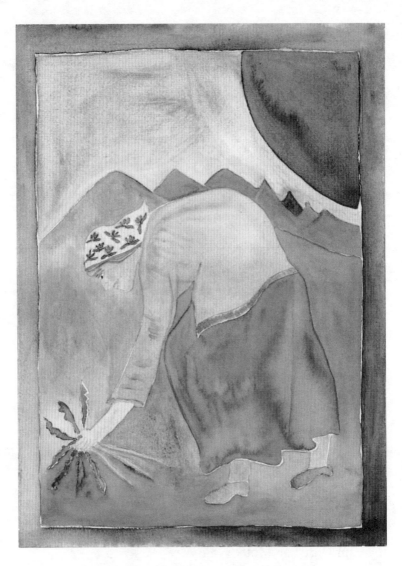

FINDING MARY

Deep in the rich dark soil of time and human culture
we will find Her roots.

"Mary has a lineage, it is more than the lineage of the House of David. All Neolithic goddess roads lead to Mary." Charlene Spretnak.

As a Catholic woman long devoted to Mary, I know my roots run deep. I have climbed aboard buses, driven in cars, walked down wide streets and through narrow cobblestone passageways alone and with other women on our way to evening prayers to her across two continents and five decades. I have been lifted up in her arms and experienced her radiant beauty firsthand. I have been consoled by her, protected by her, inspired by her and have found my refuge in her for many years.

Despite my long-standing friendship with Mary, or perhaps because of it, a book written by Charlene Spretnak, entitled *Missing Mary* had a profound effect on me. With the perspective of a scholar, Spretnak brilliantly outlines the history and culture of the Blessed Mother and delves deep into the rich soil of Mary's relationship with the church and her people. Spretnak speaks about the reemergence of Mary in today's world, which she sees as a corrective measure, bringing heart to the dominant modern, masculine mind set. This chapter, *Finding Mary*, is my direct response to *Missing Mary,* and I pay Charlene Spretnak and her work special tribute here.

Down through the millennia, since the veritable beginnings of human life and culture, countless others like us have been standing in awe of the life-giving and sustaining, nourishing, bountiful Maternal Matrix. She has been revered throughout the ages. This mother is much older than our Christian Mother Mary.

The biological processes of nature were associated with those of the human female body very early on. The ancient peoples noticed that women's menstrual cycles flowed in rhythm with the cycles of the moon and the tides of the sea. They kept track of these cycles, and so calendars and math were born. These rhythmic cycles were related to the abundance of the earth, the blessed richness and fecundity of nature. The earth produced a multitude of life forms, and provided for them all; the human female produced a living child, and nursed it at her breast with the milk produced within her own body. Both earth and female were considered sacred because of their life-sustaining nature. The life-giving, creative energy they possessed was revered.

Our Paleolithic grandmothers honored the Divine Feminine in small alcoves within their homes. By 4,400 B.C. they had elaborated a rich symbol system depicting a variety of goddesses expressing cosmological processes. They carved her likenesses in stone. They made offerings, baked cakes and burned herbs to her. They sang her praises and danced sacred dances in her name. They depended on her for their sustenance. When the waterfowl returned, and the earth greened, and food was once again abundant throughout the lands, they gave thanks to her, Great Mother of All.

By Neolithic times the Goddess's mythic presence was well established throughout all of southern and southeastern Europe as well as the Near East. Most regions had their own local goddess, or several goddesses, who expressed the unique individuality of that particular place and were seen not only as protectors of the area but also as reflecting a wide range of complex intrapersonal dynamics.

She was usually seen symbolically as a virgin, which was understood to mean that while not necessarily unacquainted with sex, she was owned by no man, she was complete, whole and independent of herself. In addition, she possessed great powers of generation and regeneration.

This Great Mother embodied the sacred whole. She was the elemental and cyclical processes of birth, maturation, death and regeneration. She was abundance. She was wisdom. She was caring, loving and just. From under the mantle of her loving protection and out of the profuse cornucopia of her bounty, came many gifts, such as the gifts of art, language, music and math. She was protector of the home and the family. She taught the people how to plant seeds and grow food; she gave us apples, olives, figs and so much more.

To be sure, not all ancient goddesses were benign, nor generous. Some were dangerous, some wrathful. For they reflected raw nature, which is sometimes to be feared. But for the most part, Great Mother was just that: Bountiful Mother of all.

She was the rolling hills and high mountains, streams, wells and springs, the lush, verdant green, the wildflowers and grains, the wild places everywhere. She was loved and revered because of her wildness and all that sprang forth from it.

"What can be said of peoples who elaborated an intimate poetic symbol of the Maternal Matrix, the life giving "plenum" from which all forms manifest and pass away in this universe, is not that they were childlike and ignorant but that they were perceptively aligning their deepest spiritual identity with the larger, profoundly relational reality, rather than holding it at arm's length, as does the ideology of both modernity and deconstructionism." Charlene Spretnak

There are many common and colorful threads clearly weaving together the myths of the ancient pre-Christian goddesses with the biblical narrative of the life of Mary.

Primeval legends tell of a goddess who gives birth to a male child parthenogenetically, by her own doing, and alternately, of a mortal woman impregnated by divine power, who produces a divine hero or demigod.

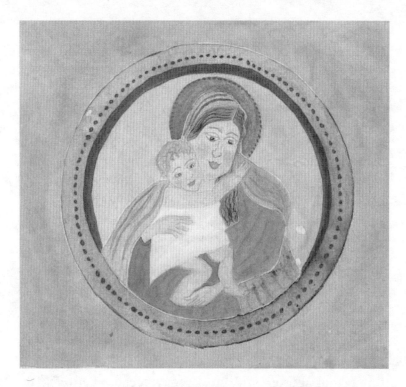

Many of the ancient goddesses were both virgin and mother, many gave birth to a son, half human, half divine, who later died and was reborn. Virgin mothers Isis, Hathor, Demeter and Cybele all followed these ancient story lines.

"In the Christian tradition the Virgin Mary is clearly rooted in the older Goddess religion because she produces her child parthenogenetically." Charlene Spretnak

Mortal Mary, impregnated by the Holy Spirit, gave birth to her divine son at the Winter Solstice; he died and was reborn at the Spring Equinox. The timing of this narrative comes to us from the earliest stirring of human cultural awareness of the changing yet constant earth. The seasonal birth, death and rebirth of the green. This story is tied to the processes of nature, the flow of the seasons, the turning of the earth and the procession of stars in the sky, the waxing and waning of the moon, the solar progression. This is an old, old story with profound cosmological proportions.

Mary and Jesus carried these most ancient story lines, these basic cosmological truths perceived and elaborated upon over thousands of years by ancient, earth-honoring peoples, woven together with their unique and timely message of love, compassion and redemption into the new era.

As we have seen, at the time of Mary and Jesus, 90 per cent of the people in the Mediterranean area were pagans whose spiritual lives and culture were informed by mythic stories of the Divine Feminine in many forms and aspects, such as protector or patron of a particular place or segment of life.

As Christianity's story of Jesus and Mary slowly spread throughout the Mediterranean area, and eventually throughout Europe, a great convergence between the Blessed Mother Mary and the local goddesses took place.

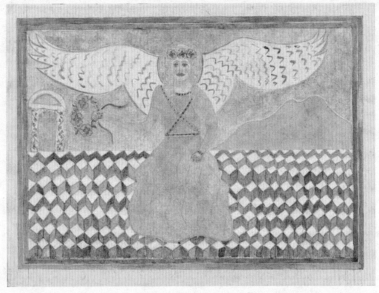

These early Christian peoples willingly embraced Mary as the new embodiment of the sacred whole, and over the ensuing centuries transferred their ages old love and devotion for the Sacred Feminine to the Blessed Mother Mary. The local forms and qualities, by which the Divine Feminine had been known, became attributes of Mary. The names and titles by which they had revered her, the ancient symbols used to depict her, the plants, animals and cosmological proportions long associated with her, were all transferred to Mary.

Queen of Heaven. Virgin of Virgins. Mother of God.

"Christianity from the very outset was a convergence of the earth honoring Motherline with the cult of the sky-god Father. The new Father-Son religion was immeasurably enriched by the compassionate and cosmological attributes of the Blessed Virgin Mary." Charlene Spretnak

Ancient symbols long associated with the Maternal Matrix were woven into the new Christian story line. The Triple Goddess, revered since remote antiquity, was known by several different names and forms throughout the Mediterranean regions, such as the three fates, and virgin, mother and crone. She was also revered as the three phases of the moon, who the Greeks called Artemis, Selene and Hecate.

The roots of the Triple Goddess go back to Paleolithic peoples for whom tri lines carved onto statuettes or painted on cave walls symbolized her presence. This ancient perception of the blessed trinity, the Triple Goddess or the sacredness of three, was absorbed into Christianity, though she was transgendered in the process. At the Council of Constantinople in 381, the doctrine of the Holy Trinity was declared, and the Father, the Son and the Holy Spirit were formally established as the defining mystery and theology of the new Christian religion.

The dove, long seen as an attribute of Venus, Goddess of Love and Beauty, now represents the Holy Spirit and is depicted suspended over Mary's head, especially in scenes of the Annunciation and Immaculate Conception. Isis, beloved by the Egyptians, Semitic peoples and the Romans, usually shown sitting on a throne with her infant son Horus in her lap, was long associated with the moon, the tides and the sea. Mary is now depicted as standing on a crescent moon, and is referred to as Star of the Sea. *Stella Maris* is a title once held by Isis.

Over the centuries, as Christianity became the main spiritual expression of the European people, the statues of Isis holding Horus were simply renamed Mary, or became the models from which new statues of Mary and the infant Jesus were created.

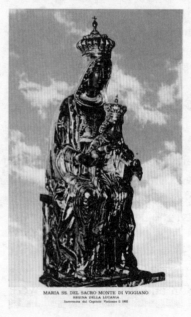

Because Isis was from Egypt, she was dark skinned, and some of these ancient renamed statues of Isis are now known as Black Madonnas, though to be certain, not all Black Madonnas were once statues of Isis. The Black Madonnas are considered to be especially powerful and great healing and fertility powers are usually attributed to them. Most of the Black Madonnas of Europe are still located in the original places where they were found, which are usually at or near ancient sites of Neolithic Goddess worship.

Many churches throughout Europe were built over these ancient Goddess sites, usually over springs or grottos or on the top of a nearby hill. These natural places were chosen because they emanated a concentrated energy field that may have enhanced the prayers and ceremonies offered there.

In Italy, churches were routinely constructed over ancient shrines once sacred to Juno, Isis, Minerva and Diana. The Basilica di Santa Maria Maggiore in Rome was constructed over an ancient temple dedicated to Cybele. The list goes on and on. In Monte San Giacomo, our church of St. James is built over an ancient spring at the very center of the village, and water flows constantly from exquisitely carved sixteenth-century marble fixtures at its side.

As we have seen, elements in the biblical story of Christ echo older and well known stories of the dying and returning gods such as Osirus, Attis, Dumuzi and Adonis. Some scholars have noted threads of the ancient story lines of Zoroaster, Dionysus, Orpheus and the Mithras cult as well within the biblical story of Jesus. And, according to Charlene Spretnak:

"It came to pass that the Last Supper was recalled in the gospels as a staging site for the appropriation of two extremely ancient sacred rituals, an absorption that must have seemed to the shapers of the Christian story as merely natural, rather than calculated. First, Christ's elevating a piece of bread and declaring "This is my body" echoes the ritual elevation of wheat in Demeter's Eleusinian Mysteries (the great initiation ritual undergone by nearly all citizens of Athens for centuries and later by many prominent Romans). The concept of Christ's being in the communion

bread also drew upon the ancient belief in Greece and several Near Eastern cultures that the Goddess of the Fruits of the Earth, including grains, was in the seed grain and in the ritual bread. According to the Christian narrative, Jesus next subsumes into his new symbol system the extremely ancient blood mysteries and rituals of the female. He elevates the wine and declares, "This is my blood." With that act, a new version of the blood mysteries is born."

And so it was that Jesus' Gospel of Love was combined with the ancient women's mysteries and thus ritually united to the primeval motherline. And is not this ancient motherline, and the profound sacred relational consciousness associated with it, reflected in the words and acts of Jesus?

"Whosoever shall humble themselves as this little child, the same is the greatest in the kingdom of heaven. And whoso shall receive one such little child in my name also receives me." Matthew 18:4-5

From where did he learn such compassion? Who taught him the blessings of forgiveness? The power of prayer? The secrets of healing? The ethical framework from which Jesus taught and operated came from deep within him and was surely influenced by his mother throughout his boyhood - as all sons are influenced by the mothers who raise them. His mother was the woman who proclaimed the Magnificat, the one with the intensely social conscience, the one who, when beckoned by an angel, agreed to give birth to the Son of God.

"His father may have been the often wrath-ful sky-god, more ancient even than Yahweh, but his mother was our Mary." Charlene Spretnak

And "our Mary"? How was *she* changed by having gestated and given birth to this Son of God? Reproductive science tells us that the cells and DNA of the baby are absorbed by its mother during its time in the womb. Science has also proven that new neural pathways are created in the mother's brain during pregnancy, childbirth and lactation. Mary has grown God in her womb, she made him from her cells, he came forth from her body, and she absorbed and took into herself parts of him. She has been changed in the same mystical way all mothers are changed after having conceived, nourished and brought forth a new life into this world. Mary is fully human and that is why we understand and resonate so deeply with her. Yet because she has given birth to God, she is also more than human. She is transcendent. She is of the earth and also of the cosmos.

The Divine presence entered into our luminous Mary at the Annunciation, and remained with her for the rest of her life on earth. Mary put a new frame around a very old story and brought the Divine Feminine securely into the Christian era entirely on her own terms.

By the magnetic, magnanimous grace of our Mary, the most ancient and primordial expressions of the Sacred Feminine have been kept alive in the West. She is our modern day Trojan Horse. Mary is the all-important vessel carrying the ancient symbols, images, celebrations, and sacred *knowings* under her skirt and behind her veil right into the midst of the twenty-first century!

Mary is lifting her skirts and throwing back her mantle now to reveal her true power, as is the ancient way of all women. The sacred secrets she has kept safely hidden there are flowing out, a rich and colorful wealth of nourishment and meaning, into our present day cultural awareness.

Mary's grace and power have not been diminished at all, not even after women's values and roles were devalued and the modern, masculine, mechanical, Newtonian world view predominated. Nor by the harsh de-throning she received at the hands of Luther and Calvin during the Protestant Reformation, when she was referred to as the "*Whore of Babylon*." Luther, admonishing his followers to rely solely on the word of God as written in the Bible, advised his congregation in 1530, to "accept the child and his birth and forget the mother."

"Defenders of the fullness of Mary's presence remind her censors that the divine plan for the salvation via the Incarnation intimately and essentially involved maternal mediation and cooperation – "the heart of a woman" – which guided the unfolding of the life of Jesus, beginning with the Annunciation." Charlene Spretnak

Mary is alive and well even after the Second Vatican Council officially reduced her role and presence in Catholic mass, life and culture in an effort to be ecumenical and reach out to their "*separated brethren.*"

In bemoaning the absence of so much of the rich heritage Catholics once embraced but that has been "pruned" from Catholic sacramental culture in recent decades, Andrew Greeley, a priest and sociologist who heads the *Recovering the Catholic Heritage* effort, wrote: *"When I am asked how the Catholic imagination differs from the Protestant, I reply that we have angels and saints and souls in Purgatory and statues and stations of the cross and votive candles and religious medals and crucifixes and rosaries and Mary the Mother of Jesus and First Communions and Candlemas and Ash Wednesday and May Crownings and midnight Masses and pilgrimages and relics – and they don't. These days I realize that we don't have most of them any more either."*

Whether or not we are Catholic, our challenge remains the same. It is to become reacquainted with the full "*biblicalplus*" spiritual presence of Mary. Each of us is called to rediscover and personally experience the richness and fecundity of her mystical dimension, her cosmological proportions. To stand firmly in the glow of her wild and compassionate heart. To bathe in the ancient, ever-flowing stream of her feminine healing grace.

This Mother Mary is here to stay. She is not going to go away. She knows us and she loves us. And we, her people, know and love her too. She is simply a part of us. She lives within our wild hearts as Mary, Mother of God, as her predecessors lived in our ancestors' hearts for more than 35,000 years of human history.

"*Our Mother Mary will not be cast down and bound up...and neither will her daughters. We will rise, daughters, we will rise.*" Sue Monk Kidd

I believe it is simply in our genetic make-up to love, revere and pay homage to our Mother. After so many years of human cultural and spiritual evolution, it must be. We have literally as well as symbolically evolved together with the Feminine Divine at the forefront of our lives and at the center of our consciousness since remotest antiquity.

Memorare: Remember, O most gracious Virgin Mary, that never was it known that anyone who fled to thy protection, implored thy help, or sought thy intercession, was left unaided.

Inspired by this confidence I fly unto thee, O Virgin of Virgins, my Mother. To thee do I come, before thee I stand, sinful and sorrowful. O Mother of the Word Incarnate, despise not my petitions, but in thy mercy hear and answer me. Amen.

"May the Blessed Virgin, Mother of Mercy, fill the hearts of all with wise thoughts and peaceful intentions."
Pope John Paul II

Pope John Paul II had a deep, lifelong devotion to Mary, Mother of God. Upon becoming pope he insisted on including a large *"M"* in his papal seal, although there was some objection to this on the part of "progressives" in the Vatican.

His papal slogan was the vow he made to Mary in his youth and kept all his life. *Totus Tuus* (My entire self is yours).

It is interesting to note that the *"M,"* which has long been used to symbolize Mary, actually has primeval roots. Marija Gimbutus tells us that the *"M"* has symbolized the presence of the Feminine Divine since the Paleolithic times.

Someone once said, and I wish I knew who so I could give them credit here: You can never entirely eliminate a stratum, you can only absorb it…and along these same lines: the past always lives on in the present.

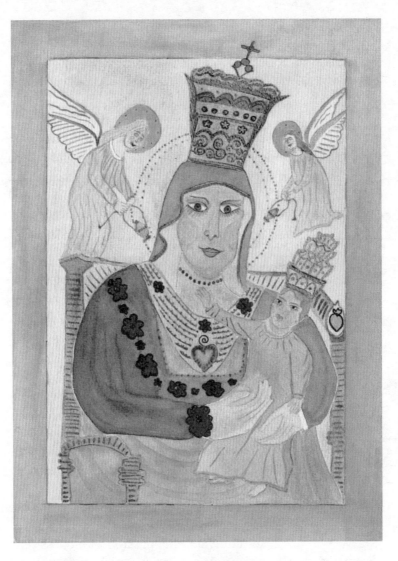

OUR WILD HEARTS AND MARY

Because our Blessed Mother Mary's roots go all the way back to primordial times and remote and ancient wild places and peoples of the earth, we can find her within our own wild places, most especially within our wild hearts.

"'Mother of God,' said August. The words hovered over us. I thought of Mary's spirit, hidden everywhere. Her heart a red cup of fierceness tucked among ordinary things. Isn't that what August had said? Here, everywhere, but hidden." Sue Monk Kidd, Secret Life of Bees

She is an integral part of us. We can find her through prayer and meditation, in a garden among her plants, deep in the woods, or high on a mountain top, wherever the earth is in her glory. We come to her through myth, prayer and metaphor, through poetry, song, ritual, dance, procession and praise. We come to her through sacred stories that have been told and retold since the beginnings of time and yet are new again with every retelling. We find her in quiet moments of repose.

Her spiritual presence can be deeply felt in meditation on the rosary and its mysteries. So much so that we learn to *"see through the eyes and heart of Mary."*

Seeing through the eyes and heart of Mary is exactly what we need to do. It is the one thing that will save the world.

Finding Mary within our wild hearts and perceiving the world "through her eyes and heart" leads to understanding the nature of compassion and to acknowledging its fundamental importance in the interrelationships of all life on earth. Perceiving the world through the wild heart of Mary, we learn to cultivate compassion, kindness and forgiveness. We begin to practice unconditional love and feel a deep sense of empathy with all of life, including ourselves. We find our true source of strength.

We become aware of an increased sense of gratitude, a renewed sense of joy and connectedness. We become naturally happier and realize why Mary has been the inspiration of artists, poets and writers throughout time and why she was chosen to be Mother of the Prince of Peace.

Our growing compassion and love for ourselves and others leads us to extend this love to all life forms on this planet from bacteria to rhinoceroses…The living earth, and all upon her, are our family.

> Since the beginning you and I have been
> Since the birth of the Universe
> we have been linked
> you and I and everything
> Our molecules
> Our chemistry
> We are metabolic exchanges
> Dancing arm in arm
> Through the ions
> playing God.

Within our communities we will see many opportunities to share and give. Doing so brings the wild heart of Mary into the communal space where it can and will be enjoyed by all. Mary is working in our hearts and through our hands, and out of the work we do in her name many blessings will flow. And peace will surely come. She has promised it.

Mary is our crossroads. She is our gateway. She is a sacred signpost leading us into the unknown territory between the ages, between old and new.

She is beyond duality. Mary speaks to us of a profound unity underlying all things and invites us to step into this sacred whole with her. This sacred relational space she has been holding through all eras…to heal…to become one with the pulsating, unified field of the millions of wild hearts beating throughout all of time who have been and are still attuned to her.

Our Mary is wild, eternal, resourceful and resilient. She shows us that all of nature is imbued with Divine presence.

"Our Lady is not some magical being out there somewhere, like a fairy godmother. She's not the statue in the parlor. She's something inside of you...When you are unsure of yourself, when you start pulling back into doubt and small living, she's the one inside saying, 'Get up from there and live like the glorious girl you are.' She's the power inside you, you understand?" Sue Monk Kidd

Communion with her, in whatever form, promotes personal and global health and leads us to the peaceful and grounded state of mind, body and society that is our natural birthright.

RECLAMATION
*It is a language lost we are talking about.
And what is necessary is a reclaiming.*

The time has come for us to reclaim an important part of our Christian story. In fact, the future of our planet and all life upon it depends on us doing so. The part we need to find, claim, develop and bring front and center, is the part that is deeply connected to nature. To woman. To the earth. To the wild heart. And that very powerful part does exist. Missing since post Medieval times perhaps, but right here nonetheless, pulsating under the surface of modern day life. Calling out to be reclaimed, retrieved, rewoven into the sacred story of life, and celebrated again, as it was in days of old.

During all the many years of evolving human culture, people learned from the open book of nature. Human beings were intimately connected to the earth, and understood her language. They did not come to this knowledge through analytical linear thinking, but through a more holistic and intuitive mode of perception. This ancient way of learning is still available to us today.

In his book, *The Secret Teachings of Plants*, Stephen Harrod Buhner tells us that all indigenous peoples say that they gained their knowledge of how to use plants as medicine from the plants themselves. They did not use trial and error, nor analytical thinking, but instead learned directly from the plants, from the living earth.

They used their wild hearts to connect to and to directly perceive the wild heart of nature.

This holistic means of cognition has not disappeared simply because left brain linear thinking is now the dominant mode of perception. This capacity to learn directly from the wild heart of nature is not limited to indigenous or ancient people. It is part of our equipment as human beings, a component of our internal structure and chemical makeup. It is still a part of who we are today and we can, with work and attention, develop this latent ability within ourselves.

"It is as natural as the beating of our hearts." Stephen Harrod Buhner

Buhner refers to this method for gathering information directly from the wild heart of nature as *biognosis* which means "knowledge from life." He says that developing this ancient mode of cognition is crucially important for us in today's world as we face many threats to the life of our planet and ourselves due to what he calls *"linear fanaticism and mechanomorphism (seeing the world as a machine)."*

Stepping into the sacred wholeness and perceiving the wild heart of nature is about much more than collecting knowledge, however. A profound *knowing* takes place; an experience and awareness of the interconnectedness of the web of life that surrounds us all.

"Redeveloping the capacity for heart-centered cognition can help each of us reclaim personal perception of the living and sacred intelligence within the world." Stephen Harrod Buhner

The Song of Songs, lyrical love poems attributed to King Solomon, but actually written down a few hundred years after he lived, were revered across Europe during Medieval times when all of nature was perceived as being imbued with Divine Presence. These Songs of Solomon come from a much earlier tradition of celebrating the human body and all of nature as holy. It is lush with the imagery of fruits and flowers, aromatic spices and trees, all of which embody the beauty of the beloved. Its poetic language celebrates the earth, her seasons, and her processes as sacred. During the Medieval times passages from these poems were applied to the Blessed Mother in liturgy and prayer. These became known as the Little Office, or Office of the Blessed Virgin Mary.

Certain lines and images in particular were drawn upon to depict Mary: *"A garden locked is my sister, my bride."* Medieval painters often painted scenes of Mary enclosed within a beautiful garden. Other images and titles inspired by these lyrical verses and associated with Mary included the sealed fountain, the Lily of the Valley, the Cedar of Lebanon and the Tower of David.

The fact that the Songs of Solomon were so revered and so widespread gives us a glimpse into the mindset of the people during these Medieval times. They were for the most part an earth-based agricultural people, wise in the ways of the earth. They possessed a knowing body. They were in tune with the earth and understood their place on it. Furthermore they perceived the cosmos as a creative unfolding, a mostly benevolent and nurturing womb.

For these people the living earth was a place of transcendent beauty and grace, and Mary, the epitome of beauty and grace, was associated with this natural world. She *was* its hills, springs and grottos. The sea and the stars.

This ancient world view of the profound interrelationship of all living beings was strongly and directly opposed by the new Abrahamic religions (Judaism, Christianity and Islam) which emphasized the word, or commandments. The struggle between these two versions of reality has gone on for millennia.

The latest science, however, especially the new physics, is proving that the reality of our Universe is more closely aligned to the ancient worldview of interconnectedness and interrelationship.

Physicists now realize that the universe is not made of matter suspended in empty space (Newtonian physics) as we have been taught, but is made of energy. Vortexes of energy, with each material structure radiating its own unique energy signature, or field. And strangely, the closer scientists are able to look at the atom, the more there is nothing to be seen. It seems that matter and energy are one and the same.

"The Universe is one indivisible, dynamic whole in which matter and energy are so deeply entangled it is impossible to consider them as separate elements." Bruce Lipton

In his book, *The Biology of Belief*, Lipton describes the universe as an integration of interdependent energy fields that are *"entangled in a meshwork of interactions with complex intercommunications among the physical parts and the energy fields that make up the whole."* He describes the flow of information in the universe as holistic and immediate, not linear. And, as far as Lipton is concerned, the mechanics of this new science reveal the existence of our spiritual essence.

His study of the single cell, which he devoted his life to understanding, brought him to the realization that just like a single cell, the character of our lives is determined by our responses to the environmental signals that propel life. His studies, he says, *"convinced me that we are immortal, spiritual beings...I realized that I could change the character of my life by changing my beliefs and thereby move from victim in the world to co-creator."*

In fact, according to Lipton, the latest discoveries in both cellular biology and physics are creating new bridges between science and spirit. *"The latest science leads us to a worldview not unlike that held by the earliest civilizations, in which every material object in Nature was thought to possess a spirit...it is the world of Gaia, a world in which the whole planet, including all the life upon it, is considered to be one living, breathing organism."*

Lipton explains that instead of trying to understand the "natural order" of things so that we could fit harmoniously into that order, the Modern Scientific movement set out on a mission of control and domination of Nature. *"The technology that has resulted from pursuing this philosophy has brought human civilization to the brink of spontaneous combustion by disrupting the web of Nature."*

Lipton concludes his book with a call to join with other like-minded people who are working toward the advancement of human civilization *"by realizing that Survival of the Most Loving is the only ethic that will ensure not only a healthy personal life but also a healthy planet."*

In much the same way that our concepts and ideas about life are ever evolving through the use of new information and associations, the same is true of earlier peoples. Much of the transfer of knowledge of Christian ideas and dogma that took place across the centuries was done simply by associating certain plants with the new biblical stories.

When early Christianity was spreading throughout the lands, itinerant priests and traveling monks used commonly found flowers and trees as teaching aids. This nature language was easily understood, and in fact, was a commonly shared knowledge among all people. These agrarian people based their plant associations on deep inherent knowledge of the plant's physical properties, its growth habit, appearance, aroma, color and form as well as its more subtle energetic qualities.

The lily, so soft and feminine yet strong and resilient, became an emblem of Mary, and associated with the Annunciation. St. John's wort, well known for its spirit healing and pain easing properties, is associated with the Passion of Jesus and the heartache of Mary. This plant oozes a red ink-like substance, very much the color of blood, when a bud or flower is squeezed between the fingers, and this led to it representing the blood of Christ.

A deep, reliable knowledge of plants existed, based on generation upon generation of using them and understanding their many gifts, both physical and energetic. This deep body of knowing acquired over many thousands of years, about nature and specifically about plants, was nearly lost during the several hundreds of years around the Protestant Reformation.

THE BURNING TIMES

After purging Europe of most of the religious heretics, the Inquisition turned its attention to "witches." During these times many people, especially women wise in the ways of healing with herbs and understanding the language of nature, faced the danger of being labeled as witches.

A lot of misinformation exists about this period of European history, sometimes referred to as the *Burning Times*. According to differing accounts, anywhere from 50,000 to as many as 9 million people, mostly women, were executed during these several hundred years. But a flood of new information on this period has been brought to light, and much of it casts serious doubt on many of the commonly held ideas about who, how many and by what means people were actually killed for being witches during this time.

To the early Christian mind, *mares, strigae* and *lamiae (night spirits)* were unsophisticated Pagan superstitions. In the early days of Christianity, the Church officially urged all Christian kings to forbid their subjects from killing women accused of being mares or witches.

The laws of the Pactus Alamannorum (613-623) created penalties for people who hung or harmed witches. The Edict of Rothari, dated 643, proclaimed it un-Christian to accuse women of such things. These laws suggest that as Christianity spread through Europe, witch hunting declined.

The Church tried most witches during the Middle Ages, and penalties were actually fairly mild. The Inquisition's job was to reconcile heretics, to bring them back into the Church. The records show that an accused witch, willing to acknowledge the *error of her ways,* was treated with considerable leniency by the Inquisitors. Few witches actually died during this period.

The worst persecutions occurred in central Europe from 1550 – 1650, during the Protestant Reformation, one of the worst periods of religious warfare Europe ever experienced. During the 16th century the rate of persecution and death skyrocketed. The witch trials dramatically decreased during the last half of the 17th century until they virtually disappeared by the end of the 18th century.

The truth is that less than 20,000 executions are recorded in Europe. As modern day historians studied the records of trial verdicts, they learned that previous estimates of the European death toll had been greatly exaggerated. Scholars are now confident that somewhere between 20,000 and 60,000 witches died during these times.

In his meticulously researched study, *Night Battles*, Carlo Ginzburg demonstrated that most Italian witches were indeed drawing on pre-Christian traditions and, like the *Good Walkers* he describes, combined both Christian and ancient shamanic beliefs which were tied to prehistoric agrarian practices.

Women made up approximately 80% of those accused of witchcraft, though this varied dramatically depending on time and place. Some northern countries put as many men as women to death, perhaps even more. In Iceland, for instance, 95% of those killed were men. But overall, far more women than men were executed, sometimes as many as 20 women for every one man.

Most of those accused as witches were poor. But in some places, especially where the witch hunter could confiscate his victim's property, accused witches are found among the wealthy as well.

A significant number of those accused were herbalists, healers and midwives. Jenny Gibbons, a scholar and historian of Medieval times and the Christian conversion of Western Europe, writes extensively on this period of history. She says that as many as one-quarter of those accused possessed knowledge of herbs and healing, or used some form of healing magic. Elderly people, unmarried, independent women and widows were assailed most frequently.

European people of the time believed they were threatened by a satanic conspiracy. Since Satan was believed to grant his followers both magical powers and great knowledge, midwives, prophets, healers, scholars and even artists could be accused of being witches. Fear of the curative powers that herbalists, healers and midwives possessed caused these skills to be demonized.

Satan was the father of heresy and encouraged all evils, especially sexual ones, so homosexuals, sexually independent and especially beautiful women and criminals all fell under suspicion. And, since all ugliness was also the work of Satan, the elderly and the physically or mentally handicapped were also suspect.

Although it is hard to believe, Gibbons explains that all segments of European society supported the witch trials. Beginning in 1022, the Church began executing those it considered heretics, people who disagreed with the core of its teachings. When the Burning Times began, Europeans had already become accustomed to burning heretics and religious dissidents.

But the Catholic Church actually killed very few witches. Most of the religious courts imposed non-lethal penalties, like penance or imprisonment. However, the Church did encourage the intolerance and stereotyping that caused the trials, and its practice of murdering dissidents laid the groundwork for executing witches.

The Inquisition played a crucial role in the persecutions by diabolizing witchcraft. But the truth is that contrary to what we've all heard, the Inquisition did not kill many witches. They *investigated* charges of witchcraft from 1300 to 1500, a time when the death rate was very low. After the Reformation, the Inquisition was quietly phased out of most European countries.

When the witch crazes swept Europe, the Inquisition existed in only two countries, Spain and Italy, both of which had exceedingly small death tolls. In fact the Spanish Inquisition killed less than 1% of those accused. In northern Italy several hundred witches were put to death, but in southern Italy there were none.

After eradicating the Cathars from France, the Inquisitors turned their attention to witches. They re-defined witchcraft as a *heresy;* it was no longer perceived as a harmless superstition requiring no punishment. Heretics were killed.

The earliest witch hunting manuals were written by inquisitors Bernard Gui, Johannes Nider and Heinrich Kramer. Kramer authored the *Malleus Maleficarum* with some help from a Dominican scholar, and this book, as well as other witch hunting manuscripts, helped to spread the fear of witchcraft throughout Europe. The *Malleus Maleficarum* has been held up as proof of the Catholic Church's lust for the murder of witches during 500 years of European history. But, according to Gibbons' extensive research, this was not the case.

Heinrich Kramer, also known as Henry Institoris, was a German Inquisitor of the late 15th century. He was not well respected and his views on witchcraft were considered both weird and extreme by most of his peers, who continually opposed and hindered his trials. Kramer conducted a large trial in Innsbruck in 1485, where 57 people were investigated. No one was convicted. The bishop of Innsbruck was so disturbed by Kramer's focus on the sexual behavior of the accused women that he closed down the trial, remarking that Satan was in the inquisitor, not the witches.

The *Malleus* is usually circulated along with the papal bull "*Summis Desiderantes,*" which rants against witches and those who oppose Kramer and his co-author, Jacob Sprenger. But Pope Innocent had not read the *Malleus* when he wrote *Summis Desiderantes*. The *Malleus* was also accompanied by a supposed recommendation from the Faculty of Cologne, the Inquisition's top theologians. Both these endorsements are misleading.

Kramer had complained to the Pope about the poor reception he was receiving from other priests, and the Pope, who greatly feared witchcraft, tried to help by giving him the Papal bull. Pope Innocent also asked a Dominican scholar, Jacob Sprenger, to help Kramer write the *Malleus*. When the writing was completed, Sprenger presented the *Malleus* to the Faculty at Cologne, asking for its approval. Instead, the Inquisition resoundingly condemned the book.

The Inquisitors stated that the procedures the book recommended were unethical and illegal, and that its demonology was totally inconsistent with Catholic doctrine. Unconcerned, Kramer forged an enthusiastic endorsement.

The Faculty quickly discovered this and was enraged. Kramer and Sprenger parted on bad terms, and the Inquisition condemned Kramer in 1490, just four years after the *Malleus* was published.

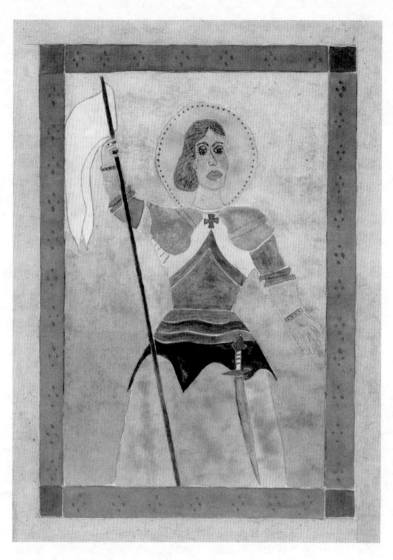

Saint Joan of Arc Though quite accomplished at feminine skills such as sewing and embroidery, Joan of Arc preferred the life of a soldier. Passionate that France not be lost to the English, Joan donned masculine attire and convinced the King to let her lead the battle in defense of France. A heroine when good fortune led to success for the French forces, Joan lost the good will of her supporters when she fell in battle. She was burned at the stake as a heretic and fifty years later was proclaimed a saint.

It was not the Catholic Church, but actually the secular governments who did most of the killing during these times. In fact, it was the fortunate witch who was tried by the Church. The death toll was always lowest when and where the Church ran the trials, and their courts usually killed less than 1% of the people they tried. The truly damned were tried by the secular courts. They tried far more witches than the religious courts did; the records show that most of the great witch crazes and trials were carried out by secular officials. These local, secular tribunals were often no more than slaughter houses, and as many as 90% of those tried by these courts were killed.

Documents show that most of the intellectuals of the time not only accepted, but openly supported the persecutions. In fact, after the 15th century, witch hunting manuals were being written by secular intellectuals. These manuals, and vivid descriptions of the trials, were among the earliest and by far the most popular books printed in England.

Peasants were also active participants in the trials. They initiated most of the trials and were usually the main witnesses against the accused. Lynching and vigilantism were common and suspected witches were often brutalized; to break a supposed *curse,* people slashed an alleged witch's face with a knife. They murdered witches' *familiars*, threw rocks at their homes and held their heads underwater until they promised to remove a *hex*. And when a professional healer couldn't cure a disease, he or she often blamed the sickness on a witch.

For insight into this period of history and the dynamics of the witch trials, consider visiting Jenny Gibbons' extensive website: www.summerlands.com/crossroads/remembrance

I also highly recommend the play *Saint Joan of Arc* by George Bernard Shaw.

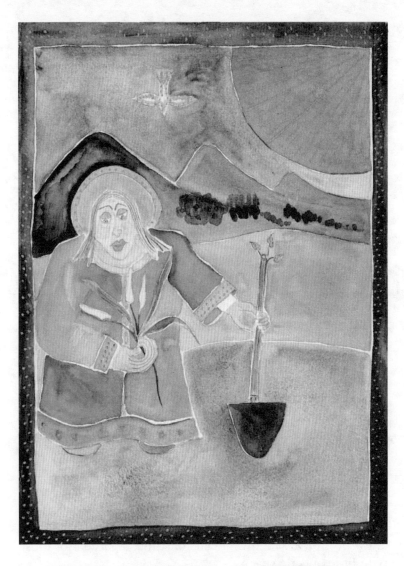

THE MARY GARDEN

Because of the intense fear of witches and all things pagan, folk wisdom and shamanic practices associated with plants, healing and nature became suspect. This great body of knowledge, the wisdom accrued over millennia regarding the healing properties of the wondrous earth and of herbs, flowers and trees was forced underground. Under the surface. It was hidden and for the most part, forgotten. But it certainly was not, nor could it ever be, lost.

This knowledge of the plants, of the earth and all of nature and its ways, is inherent wisdom. It comes with our humanness. It is part of our genetic makeup as beings of this planet. It is the fruit of inter-communication between humans and plants.

This is the wisdom of our cells, formed over eons of co-evolution with all the other life forms on our earth. This is the wisdom of life itself living within us. We can trust it. We need only remember.

There are many ways to do this. One way to remember is through contemplation on nature - in wild and natural places, or in the cultivation of a sacred garden space.

Another is through meditation on the mysteries of the rosary, once known as the Angelic Psalter, and the plants long associated with each of these sacred stories. I want to focus on these two approaches here.

Gardeners have always been aware of the spiritual element in planting and caring for plants in a garden. A garden is a transcendent place, one that reveals many spiritual lessons over time that apply to all other aspects of our lives. Even a few pots on a windowsill can constitute a garden for those with little outside space.

Among gardeners with a devotion to Mary, there is a blossoming movement called the Mary Garden. A Mary Garden is composed entirely of plants dedicated to Mary, by name, legend or history. Creating and tending a Mary Garden combines a gardener's reverence for the Blessed Mother with the love of plants and flowers. The name

"Mary Garden" stems from medieval religious art depicting the Virgin and Child in an enclosed garden amidst symbolic flowers.

Attending to a sacred growing place provides the gardener with opportunities for sacramental encounter. And since at least the Medieval times, there has been a celebrated relationship between flowers and gardens dedicated to Mary, Mother of God.

Most of what we know of Medieval gardens is of the herb and vegetable gardens meticulously cultivated by monastic groups. St. Benedict is known to have cultivated a rose garden, or "rosary," way back in the fourth century. The first garden known to be dedicated to the Blessed Mother is the one planted by St. Fiacre, the Irish patron saint of gardening. St. Fiacre cultivated his Mary Garden at the hospice he built for the poor and infirm in France during the seventh century.

In the early days of European Christianity, most of the faithful were illiterate peasants who worked closely with the earth through the seasons. They were deeply in tune with the earth, understood the language of nature and learned directly from her, by means and interactions that we would call *shamanic* today.. They developed wisdom and knowledge and grew spiritually through the imagery inspired by the earth, such as a fertile valley, hills, running springs and especially through flowers, plants and trees. These images inspired by nature found their way into the grandest of cathedrals and religious art.

The early Church teachers, such as St. Francis of Assisi, 1181-1226, used flowers as a kind of text book to help explain the mysteries, stories and teachings of Christ, the Blessed Mother and all the saints as they went about preaching.

As Christianity spread and missionaries traveled into new lands, it was rightly perceived as unwise to attempt to eradicate all of the customs and rites of the pagan religions. Even the Romans did not do this. Instead they allowed people in their conquered lands to continue their individual rites and customs, while offering them increased economic and social opportunities (as long as they were cooperative).

Some of these ancient seasonal rites, developed and celebrated for thousands of years by earth-based agricultural peoples, were enacted to ensure the cohesiveness of the community. These seasonal celebrations and the plants associated with them were easily integrated into the church's evolving liturgy and rites, and it made perfect sense to relate the emerging Christian story to these ancient seasonal celebrations. Thus the holly and the Yule log, as well as the sacred fir tree, long associated with Druid winter rites, became important themes in Christian Nativity festivals among northern Europeans.

The pre-Christian peoples had dearly loved gods and goddesses to whom they made votive offerings, presented petitions and courted favor. Jupiter, Venus, Diana, Isis, Hera, Hora, Ashtart, Cybele and Demeter, Ceres, Pan, Athena, Daphne, Adonis and many others were worshiped publicly in magnificent temples placed in the midst of beautifully manicured expanses, such as the ones that are nearly perfectly preserved in Paestum, Herculeum and Pompeii.

These gods and goddesses also had small altars dedicated to them inside of every home, as can clearly be seen in the excavations of Pompeii. Slowly, over the ensuing centuries, Christianity, and the figures it revered, became dominant. Venus, Isis and Diana bowed before the presence of Mary, and Mary openly absorbed into her persona all that had previously been attributed to them, including the flowers associated with them throughout the preceding millennia.

This evolutionary process happened many times with flowers and plants. Many plants that had previously been devoted to the goddesses worshiped by earth-honoring peoples carried names reflecting this. For instance, the well known Maidenhair fern was known in Iceland as *Freyje's Hair*. Its botanical name, *Adiantum capillus-veneris*, tells us that it was later considered sacred to Venus. We know it now as a plant dedicated to Mary.

Our Lady opened up her arms, spread wide her cloak and absorbed them all. Plants sacred to Venus, or her Scandinavian counterpart, Freyje, or to some other great female divinity, slowly became associated with Mary, mother of Jesus. Plants long associated with Juno, Diana, Hulda and Bertha became Our Lady's plants. The anemone, poppy and violet, dedicated to Venus, and the willow once sacred to Ceres, are all considered plants of Mary now.

Calendula is the first flower known to actually be named in honor of Mary. It is said that St. Hildegard of Bingen dedicated calendula to Mary and gave it the name *Mary's Gold* after having a vision. A recipe written in 1373 calls for "*seint mary gouldes*" to create a tonic to help ward off the plague. *Our Lady's Slipper* is mentioned in the herbal of Vitus Auslasser published in Germany in 1479.

During the Reformation plant names evolved again to reflect the new Protestant movement away from "worship" of Our Lady. Herbs and flowers with names such as Lady, Lady's and Ladies are considered by most authorities to be older English plant names that once referred to Mary and became more generic during this period so as to describe any woman. The plant we now know as Lady's Mantle was once called Our Lady's Mantle.

Hundreds of plants can be used to create your own Mary Garden and most are easy to grow or easy to find at any garden centre. They include the marigolds, or *Mary's gold*, the mayflower, or *Mary's flower*, and thrift, known as *Our Lady's pin cushion*. Canterbury bells are called *Our Lady's nightcap* because they look like an old-fashioned nightcap, and Fuchsia is called *Our Lady's eardrops* because the flowers resemble pendant earrings.

Several plants whose leaves are white-spotted are said in popular legends to have derived their spots from drops of the Virgin's milk that fell on them. Among these are Our Lady's thistle, virgin's thistle, lady's milk or holy thistle, all names for the same plant, commonly called milk thistle (*Silybum marianum*).

Two flowers, above all others, are emblematic of the Blessed Virgin. They are the rose and the lily. At the Feast of the Visitation (July 2), commemorating the visit of Mary to her cousin Elizabeth, the Madonna Lily (*Lilium candidum*) is a symbol of Mary's virginity, and almost all art depicting this visit has a vase of these lilies, usually with three blossoms, included. The pure white sepals are said to represent Mary's body and the golden anthers her soul, sparkling with divine light.

Roses, sacred to Venus, Diana and Aphrodite since the most ancient times, became known as the *Emblem of Mary* in the dawning Christian era. Mary is also known as the Mystical Rose. According to a well-known legend, St. Thomas, not believing the reports about the resurrection of the Virgin, had her tomb opened. Inside, instead of her body, he found the tomb filled with lilies and roses.

> *O Mary we crown thee with blossoms today*
> Queen of the angels, queen of the May...

The verdant month of May has been dedicated to Mary in honor of her fecundity since it was first proclaimed so in Naples during the 18th century. The idea quickly spread throughout the Catholic world. I remember well the lovely processions we participated in each May in honor of Mary throughout my childhood in Catholic school. Though the statue of Mary is still crowned with a wreath of fresh flowers in many European countries, this lovely devotional custom, with ancient roots, has mostly died out in the United States and other "progressive" countries since the Second Vatican Council of the 1960s. You might consider reviving this beautiful tradition within your family or community as a way of stimulating the association between nature and spirituality.

May comes from the name of the Greek nymph *Maia*, mother of Hermes with Zeus, who together with her sisters, was turned into the constellation Pleiades. These seven stars, or sisters, appear in the sky during the month of May, announcing the coming of summer's fruitfulness.

May was sacred to Flora, the Roman goddess of flowers and of spring, who was celebrated each year during *Ludi Floreales* from late April into early May. Flora was especially associated with the May blossom, or hawthorn tree. Well into the medieval times, people still honored the pagan Queen of May, who often married the Green Man in spring festivals.

What follows is an inventory of plants suitable for planting in a Mary Garden. They are listed by their common name first, followed by their Latin name and then their traditional spiritual or religious name. This list is by no means complete.

Annual and Perennial flowers for your Mary Garden:

Common Name	Botanical Name	Spiritual Name
Anemone	*Anemone nemorosa*	Flowers of the Field
Angel's Trumpet	*Datura spp.*	Beautiful Lady
Baby's Breath	*Gypsophila paniculata.*	Our Lady's Veil
Bethlehem Star	*Ornithogalum umbellatum.*	Mary's Tears
Bleeding Heart	*Dicentra spectabilis*	Mary's Heart
Bluets	*Houstonia caerul.*	Madonna's Eyes
Buttercup	*Ranunculus acris*	Lady's Locks
Canterbury Bells	*Campanula medium*	Mary Bells
Carnation	*Dianthus caryophy.*	Mary's Love of God
Castor Bean	*Ricinus communis*	Christ's Palm
Clematis	*Clematis vitalba*	Our Lady's Bower
Columbine	*Aquilegia vulgaris*	Lady's Shoes
Cornflower	*Centaurea cyanus*	Mary's Crown
Forget-me-not	*Myosotis alpestris*	Eyes of Mary
Foxglove	*Digitalis purpurea*	Virgin's Glove
Fuchsia	*Fuchsia hybrida*	Lady's Eardrops
Gladiolas	*Gladiolus spp.*	Ladder to Heaven
Globe Amaranth	*Gomphrena globosa*	Christ's Cloak
Heather	*Calluna vulgaris*	Our Lady's Adversary
Hollyhock	*Althea rosea*	St. Joseph's Staff
Honeysuckle	*Lonicera caprifolium*	Lady's Fingers
Impatiens	*Impatiens wallerana*	Mother Love
Jasmine	*Jasminum sp.*	Mary
Job's Tears	*Coix lacryma-jobi*	Mary's Tears, Rosary
Ladyslipper	*Paphiopedilum*	Lady's Slipper
Larkspur	*Delphinium ajacis*	Mary's Tears
Love-in-a-Mist	*Nigella damascena*	Lady in the Shade
Marigold	*Calendula officinalis*	Mary's Gold
Monkshood	*Aconitum napellus*	Mary's Slipper
Morning Glory	*Ipomoea purpurea*	Our Lady's Mantle
Nasturtium	*Tropaeolum majus*	St. Joseph's Flower
Pansy	*Viola tricolor*	Mary's Delight
Pearly Everlasting	*Anaphalis margarit.*	Our Lady Never Fade
Peony	*Paeonia officinalis*	Mary's Rose
Periwinkle	*Vinca minor*	Virgin Flower
Petunia	*Petunia hybrida*	Our Lady's Praises
Philodendron	*Philodendron spp.*	Holy Spirit Plant
Primrose	*Primula vulgaris*	Lady's Frills
Sea Lavender	*Limonium vulgare*	Lady's Flower
Snapdragon	*Antirrhinum magus*	Infant Jesus' Shoes

Soapwort	*Saponaria officinalis*	Lady by the Gate
Touch-Me-Not	*Impatiens capensis*	Lady's Earrings
Sweet Alyssum	*Alyssum maritimum*	Flower of the Cross
Sweet Scabious	*Scabiosa atropurpurea*	Mary's Pincushion
Sweet Pea	*Lathyrus odoratus*	Our Lady's Sweet Pea
Sweet William	*Dianthus barbatus*	Lady Tuft
Tobacco	*Nicotiana tabacum*	Holy Herb
Water Lily	*Nymphaea alba*	Lady of the Lake
Wisteria	*Wisteria frutescens*	Virgin's Bower
Zinnia	*Zinnia spp.*	The Virgin

Bulbs:

Hyacinths – symbolize the desire for peace and are dedicated to Mary
Madonna Lily – symbolizes Mary's purity, motherhood and peace.
Yellow Flag Iris – the fleur-de-lis –symbol of Mary's suffering during the Passion
Tulips – Mary's Prayer
Daffodils – Mary's Star

Specific varieties include:

Hyacinth	*Hyacinthus oriental*	Lily-of-Valley
Poet's Narcissus	*Narcissus poeticus*	Lady's Rose
Daffodil	*Narcissus pseudo N.*	Mary's Star
Polyanthus Narcissus	*Narcissus tazetta*	Rose of Sharon
Angel's Tears	*Narcissus triandrus*	Angel's Tears
Red Lily	*Lilium bulbiferum*	Mary's Lily
Madonna Lily	*Lilium candidum*	Virgin Lily
Easter Lily	*Lilium longiflorum*	Easter Lily
Mary Iris	*Iris barnumae*	Mary Iris
Madonna Iris	*Iris florentina*	Madonna Iris
German Iris	*Iris germanica*	Mary's Sword of
Ave Maria Iris	*Iris germanica*,var	Ave Maria
Moonlight Madonna	*Iris germanica*,var.	Moonlight Madonna
Yellow Flag	*Iris pseudacorus*	Emblem of Mary

Medicinal and culinary herbs for your Mary Garden:

Angelica	*Angelica archangelica*	Angels Herb
Anise	*Pimpinella anisum*	Our Lady's Tobacco
Basil	*Ocimum basilicum*	Holy Communion Basil
Bee-Balm	*Monarda didyma*	Sweet Mary
Blessed Thistle	*Cnicus benedictus*	Our Lady's Thistle
Blue Cohosh	*Caulophyllum thal.*	Our Lady's Root
Boneset	*Eupatorium perfoliatum*	Mary

Catnip	*Nepeta cataria*	Mary's Nettle
Chamomile	*Matricaria officinalis*	Mary's Plant
Chicory	*Cichorium intybus*	Heavenly Way
Coltsfoot	*Tussilago farfara*	So Before the Father
Fennel	*Foeniculum vulgare*	Lady's Fennel
Fenugreek	*Trigonella foeniculum*	Beautiful Mary
Feverfew	*Chrysanthemum parthen.*	Mary's Flower
Goldenrod	*Solidago spp.*	Our Lady's Plant
Horehound	*Marrubium vulgare*	Mother of God's Tea
Lady's Mantle	*Alchemilla vulgaris*	Our Lady's Mantle
Lavender	*Lavandula officinalis*	Our Lady's Drying Herb
Lemon Balm	*Melissa officinalis*	Sweet Mary
Lily-of-Valley	*Convallaria majalis*	Our Lady's Tears
Lovage	*Levisticum officinalis*	Our Lady's Duster
Marjoram	*Origanum vulgaris*	Our Lady's Bedstraw
Marshmallow	*Althea officinalis*	Our Lady's Cheeses
Meadowsweet	*Filipendula spp.*	Our Lady of the Meadow
Milk Thistle	*Silybum Marianum*	Our Lady's Milk Thistle
Mints	*Mentha spp.*	Mary's Bitter Sorrow
Motherwort	*Leonurus cardiaca*	Mary's Hand
Mullein	*Verbascum thapsus*	Mary's Candle
Passion Flower	*Passiflora incarnata*	Flower-of-Cross
Poppy	*Papaver rhoeas*	Christ's Blood
Red Clover	*Trifolium pratense*	Our Lady's Posies
Roses	*Rosa spp.*	Our Lady's Emblem
Rosemary	*Rosmarinus officinalis*	Rose of Mary
Rue	*Ruta graveolens*	Herb of Grace
Sage	*Salvia officinalis*	Mary's Shawl
Self-Heal	*Prunella vulgaris*	Lady's Tresses
Shepard's Purse	*Capsella bursa-pastoris*	Lady's Pouches
St. John's wort	*Hypericum perforatum*	Mary's Tears/Glory
Solomon's Seal	*Polygonatum officinale*	Mary's Seal
Speedwell	*Veronica officinalis*	Our Lady's Resting Place
Tansy	*Tanacetum vulgare*	Jesus wort/Our Lady's Plant
Thyme	*Thymus vulgaris*	The Virgin's Humility
Valerian	*Valeriana officinalis*	Our Lady's .Needlework
Vervain	*Verbena officinalis*	Herb of the Cross
Violet	*Viola odorata/alba*	Mary's Humility/Delight
Wormwood	*Artemisia absinthia*	Mary's Tree

Trees for your Mary Garden:

Almond	*Prunus amygdalus*	Symbol: Virgin Birth
Apple	*Malus sylvestris*	Mary's Apple

Apricot	*Prunus armeniaca*	Eden Apples
Arborvitae	*Thuja occidentalis*	Tree of Life
Avocado	*Persea americana*	Holy Ghost Pear
Balm of Gilead	*Populus candicans*	Balm of Gilead
Birch, White	*Betula papyrifera*	Our Lady of the Woods
Cacao	*Theobroma cacao*	God's Tree
Cherry	*Prunus avium*	Flight out of Egypt
Fig	*Ficus petiolaris*	Mary's Tree
Frangipani	*Plumeria rubra*	Mary's Flower
Ginkgo	*Ginkgo biloba*	Maiden's Hair
Hawthorn	*Crataegus spp.*	Mary's Mayflower
Lemon	*Citrus limonia*	Symbol: Mary's Fidelity
Lime	*Citrus aurantifolia*	Adam's Apple
Lombardy Poplar	*Populus nigra*	Our Lady's Poplar
Norfolk Pine	*AraucarIa excelsa*	Christmas Tree Plant
Orange	*Citrus sinensis*	Symbol: Mary's Purity
Pear	*Pyrus communis*	Mary's Fruitfulness
Pine Tree	*Pinus halapensis*	Hand of Christ
Plum	*Prunus domestica*	Mary's Plum
Pomegranate	*Punica granatum*	Mary's Virtues
Quaking Aspen	*Populus tremuloides*	Symbol: The Cross
Sycamore	*Ficus sycomorus*	Mary's Tree
Willow	*Salix alba*	Flight out of Egypt

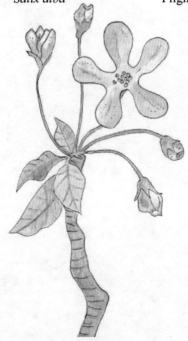

> "The Rosary is a blessed blending of mental and vocal prayer by which we honor and learn to imitate the mysteries and the virtues of the life, death, passion and glory of Jesus and Mary."
>
> St. Louis De Montfort

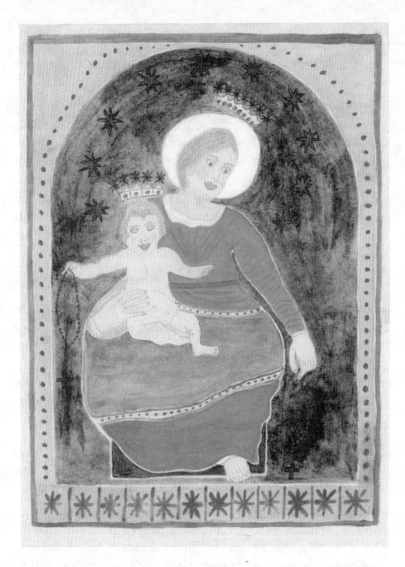

THE ANGELIC PSALTER

The rosary is a string of beads used as an implement of prayer and meditation. It is also a powerful tool for peace.

It's devotional use combines both vocal and mental prayer. The vocal prayer of the rosary consists of five decades of

Hail Marys with each decade headed by one Our Father. The mental prayer consists of contemplation on each sacred mystery as it is presented at the beginning of the decade.

The rosary prayers are the two oldest prayers in the Christian tradition and come to us directly from the life and times of Jesus and Mary. They are composed of the simple prayer that Jesus taught us when asked by a disciple, *"Lord, teach us to pray,"* and the Angelic Salutation as it was offered to Mary by the angel Gabriel. These two simple prayers likely represent the first communal devotional prayer of the early apostles, and their use has steadily continued down through the centuries. The rosary is in essence an ancient gospel prayer.

The rosary prayers combine the core of the teachings of the fatherline, as distilled through the mind and heart of Jesus, with the teachings of the motherline and all of its primordial truth and beauty. The rosary, and its mysteries, are a coalescence of the yin and yang of our Christian identity. They reveal the true mother/father heart of our Christian experience. They emphasize and help us to realize the basic underlying unity of all life, even within seeming polarity.

No one really knows how long people have been using beads for prayer. But the association is ancient among the Hindus in India, who are the first people recorded to use prayer beads, or *malas*. Their Goddess of Wisdom, Sarasvati, is very closely associated with this circle of 108 prayer beads. She is depicted holding them in one of her four hands, indicating her role as inspiration for those engaged in spiritual practice.

The Hindus are believed to have passed the practice on to the Buddhists in Tibet and China, who kept this good thing going in Japan.

The Muslims also use beads to recite the ninety nine names of Allah. Some scholars suggest that the practice of using beads to pray was brought back to the West by Crusaders who came in contact with it in the Holy Lands. By the Middle Ages prayer beads were widely in use among all strata of European people.

Prayer beads have been made out of many materials, such as wood, seeds, flower resins, semiprecious jewels and simple ropes with knots in place of beads. *"Beads have been worn around the neck, around the wrist, around the finger, and around the waist, as well as in headdresses and breastplates and in many other ways. And always they are used for spiritual and prayerful purposes."* M. Basil Pennington, Praying by Hand

The rosary had clearly been in use for centuries as a way of prayer before it was established in the year 1207 as we know it today. Legend has it that Our Lady appeared to St. Dominick and gave him the modern rosary. According to the story related by Blessed Alan De Roche, Mary referred to the string of prayer beads as her *Angelic Psalter*, called it an instrument of peace, and said that its mysteries were the foundation of the New Testament.

In 1250 Thomas of Contimpre referred to this string of beads as a *rosarium*, or rose garden. This image of the rosary, as so many roses being offered as gifts to Our Lady, took root. The rosary has been associated with this image ever since.

When the Blessed Mother appeared to three children at Fatima, Portugal, in the early years of the twentieth century, she had a long rosary hung over her arm. Mary prayed with the children and taught Jacinta, one of the three, how to properly pray the rosary.

Mary called on everyone to say the rosary daily for peace on earth and the end of all war. At her last apparition at Fatima Mary declared: ***"I am the Lady of the Rosary. Continue to say the rosary every day."***

In the apparitions of the Blessed Mother that continue to take place in Medugorje, Yugoslavia, Mary implores us to pray the rosary. And she asks us to pray from our hearts.

The Ave Maria prayer, or Hail Mary, makes it easy to do this. It is a simple, potent and beautiful prayer. The angelic salutation, as it is also known, is a concise summary of all that Catholic theology teaches about the Blessed Virgin Mary. The prayer is divided into two parts: the first part is praise, and comes directly from the words spoken by the angel Gabriel to Mary. The second part is a petition that was added later, its wording canonized by Pope Saint Pius V in 1568.

**Hail Mary, full of grace, the Lord is with thee.
Blessed art thou among women,
and blessed is the fruit of thy womb, Jesus.**

**Holy Mary, Mother of God
pray for us
now and at the hour of our death. Amen**

"By the angelic salutation God became man, a virgin became the Mother of God and the souls of the just were delivered." St. Louis De Montfort, *The Secret of the Rosary.*

The other major prayer of the rosary, the Our Father, or Lord's Prayer, is felt to be a condensation of all the beautiful sayings of the Psalms and Canticles and a summary of the whole gospel. It was given to us directly by Jesus when he taught us how to pray in his Sermon on the Mount. This is the prayer that Jesus asked us to recite:

**Our Father who art in heaven hallowed be thy name.
Thy kingdom come, they will be done
on earth as it is in heaven.
Give us this day our daily bread
and forgive us our trespasses
as we forgive those who trespass against us
and lead us not into temptation
but deliver us from evil. Amen**

These two simple and ancient prayers form the heart and soul of the rosary. Repeating these uncomplicated, trance-inducing prayers allows us to enter into deep communion and contemplation of each mystery. With these easy and straightforward words, we step effortlessly into the timeless sacred dance of our ancestors.

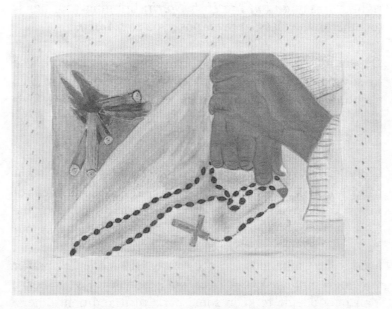

HOW TO PRAY THE ROSARY

Holding the rosary in your hands you will see a cross, followed by a singular bead, followed by three beads and another singular bead. A small triangle unites these beads to a circle of fifty-five beads.

Catholics make the sign of the cross before beginning the rosary. Crossing oneself is an ancient protective practice and far predates Christian prayer life. It was adopted by Christians as a form of protection during prayer and a way of creating sacred space. This simple ritual conveys to the mind that it is now time for prayer.

The prayer of the Trinity, the central mystery of Christian faith, goes along with the sign of the cross. Bringing the fingers of your right hand to your forehead you say **In the name of the Father**; bringing your fingers to the center of your chest, near the heart, you say **and of the Son**; bringing your hands first to the left shoulder and then crossing to the right, you say **and of the Holy Spirit;** bringing your hands together in the classic prayer pose you say **Amen.**

Depending on your own personal beliefs you may choose to say Maiden, Mother, Crone instead of the traditional Catholic blessing, or say or do something else that feels good to you, or nothing at all. This is your prayer time. You can organize it any way you want to.

Catholics say an opening prayer as we hold the cross in our hand following the sign of the cross. It is our statement of faith. This prayer is the ancient baptismal symbol of the Church of Rome. For each of us, depending on our personal beliefs, this prayer may be different. One does not need to be Catholic to say the rosary. This opening prayer may be eliminated if it does not resonate in your heart. You may decide to keep some parts of it and omit others. What follows is the traditional prayer of the Catholic Church, called the Apostles' Creed:

I believe in God, our Father Almighty *(Here I say father/mother almighty because Pope John Paul II said that God could be considered female, and that it was acceptable to refer to God as our mother as well as our father. These open and accommodating views of his are, of course, what endeared Pope John Paul II to people all over the world).* **Creator of heaven and earth and in Jesus Christ his only Son, our Lord, who was conceived by the Holy Spirit, born of the Virgin Mary, suffered under Pontius Pilate, was crucified, died and was buried. He descended into hell. The third day he rose again from the dead. He ascended into heaven and sits at the right hand of the father. From thence he shall come to judge the living and the dead. I believe in the Holy Spirit, the holy catholic Church, the communion of saints, the forgiveness of sins, and in life everlasting. Amen.**

One then proceeds by saying the Lord's Prayer on the first bead, three Hail Marys, one on each of the three beads that follow (These three beads can be seen as analogous of the three Marys, the three fates or the mystery of the Triple Goddess or Holy Trinity.), and the Lord's Prayer again on the last of the opening beads. On this last bead one also announces the first mystery. If we are meditating on the Joyful mysteries, then we say *The Annunciation* here. We spend a few moments meditating on this mystery, and then begin saying a Hail Mary on each of the ten beads that follow. This constitutes the first decade.

As we say the Hail Marys, our mind stays focused on the sacred mystery, following its implications, and perhaps receiving insights. When we reach the solitary bead that begins the second decade, we say the Lord's Prayer, announce the second Joyful mystery, *The Visitation,* meditate on its meaning for a few moments, and then go on to say the next ten Hail Marys while meditating on the second mystery.

We continue in this way around the beads, until we've recited five decades. Upon completion of the five decades we are said to have created a crown of roses for Our Lady. When we reach the little triangle connecting the circle, we say the Hail Holy Queen, or Salve Regina.

This is a very beautiful and soul nourishing prayer that is dear to my heart. The Salve Regina was recited at the end of every mass when I was a child, in honor of the Blessed Mother. The Second Vatican Council in the 1960s brought an end to this Marian devotion. Such a shame…

Hail Holy Queen was written in the ninth century by a monk named Herman, and it became the favorite song of monks everywhere. This plaintive, evocative plea to Our Lady was soon adopted as the conclusion for the rosary.

Hail Holy Queen, Mother of Mercy
Our life our sweetness and our hope,
To thee do we cry, poor banished children of Eve
To thee do we send up our sighs,
mourning and weeping in this valley of tears.
Turn then, most gracious advocate,
thine eyes of mercy toward us;
and after this, our exile,
show unto us the blessed fruit of thy womb, Jesus.

Oh clement, oh loving, oh sweet Virgin Mary.

There are two more prayers you may decide to use. One, called the Doxology, honors the mystery of the Holy Trinity and is usually recited on the same beads as the Lord's Prayer, and said directly after:

Glory be to the Father and to the Son and to the Holy Spirit, as it was in the beginning, is now and ever shall be, world without end. Amen.

The other prayer is one that the Blessed Mother is supposed to have given the children at Fatima, asking that they add it to their rosary prayers. It too is usually said on the Lord's Prayer bead.

Oh my Jesus, forgive our sins, protect us from hell, lead all souls to heaven, especially those most in need of your mercy.

The rosary and its four sets of five mysteries have a flow. This flow reminds me quite a bit of the I Ching, the Chinese Book of Changes. The 20 mysteries of the rosary take us through the evolution of the life of Christ through the eyes and heart of Mary. Mary and Jesus are perceived as a spiritual pair, a symbolic unity with extremely ancient resonance. Saying the rosary as a daily spiritual practice and meditating on the cycles of the mysteries is simply a beautiful, long appreciated way to open one's heart. To soften one's heart.

We step into each of these sacred mysteries as if it were a mythic ritual performance unfolding before our eyes. We become the players, we feel the feelings and we participate in the drama. Each mystery is multivalent and meditation on it may take us on a journey to a new destination or present us with a new insight. The unfolding of the mysteries is cyclic, we return again and again over time to the same mystery, on each occasion going deeper.

There are twenty mysteries. The five Joyful mysteries take us through the magical becoming of Christ along with Mary. The five Luminous Mysteries focus on the life of Jesus and the work he did. In the five Sorrowful Mysteries we share the depth of Christ's sorrow through the eyes of his mother. The five Glorious mysteries bring us back to life and hope. The mysteries represent the complete cycle of life, growth, death and renewal. They tell a primeval story.

These mysteries link us with the timelessness of the earth and with earth's processes as well. They link us to much older, more ancient mysteries, those celebrated by people long before Christianity, Christ and Mary.

The stories of the ancients were stories based on the poetic theological truths revealed to them through participation in cosmological life processes. Basic truths. The truths of the workings of the universe. The sacred unfolding of the story of Mary and Jesus was overlaid on the rich fabric of these more ancient earth-sky-moon-star stories until what has emerged is a sacred mythic story containing all the elements of the oldest, most basic, universal truths. Yet this story is uniquely new and true to itself in every way.

The rosary mysteries focus our minds and hearts on the story of our birth as a Christian people, as a culture. The mysteries, and the simple prayers said between each one, speak an easy, poetic language of imagery that frees the logical mind and stimulates the intuitive/insightful processes. Those knowledgeable in prayer and contemplation say that there are three ways to pray the rosary. One feature common to all of them is the interior prayer of the heart.

The simplest way to pray the rosary is to merely hold it in one's hand, to simply be with the rosary in a reverent and prayerful way, perhaps in deep contemplation with Mary on the face of Christ, or on one of the 20 mysteries. This is called the contemplative approach.

and Mary pondered all these things in her heart...

The literal or vocal approach means to say the rosary prayers while focused on the words and meanings of the prayers which spring from our personal faith.

In the meditative approach we stop at the announcement of each new mystery and meditate on it for a few moments as we've discussed above. Meditation engages our thought, imagination, emotion and desire and is a necessary step to union with the Divine. I've found it very helpful in my own practice to have a visual image in my mind that is associated with each mystery. You may choose to use the images presented here or find others that resonate in your heart. The literal and meditative approaches work very well together.

An important thing to know about the rosary is that you need to develop a practice. Saying the rosary is participatory. It is powerful. And its fruits are cumulative. In many ways developing a rosary practice is about stepping into a community of sacred space held by millions of other hearts who are also praying the rosary, and all those who have prayed the rosary throughout time. This sacred circle gets bigger and gains more momentum with every rosary recitation. One day our prayers will reach a critical mass and suddenly everything will shift. We will have grounded world peace. Mary says we can do it.

In her book *The Millionth Circle,* Jean Shinoda Bolen discusses this concept and its repercussions. *"The millionth circle depends upon a simple hypothesis, whose mechanism has already been proposed and observed, and is one that can be intuitively grasped: when a critical number of people change how they think and behave, the culture will also, and a new era begins."*

Once these principles are understood, then recitation of the rosary can be seen as an exceedingly powerful, revolutionary, evolutionary movement hidden in plain sight - a movement that can and will advance societal and global progress toward world peace.

I encourage you to set aside a special time and place for saying the rosary each day. Or during the middle of each night. If you are one of those people who find themselves lying awake at night, take your rosary in hand. Repetition of the simple prayers and the comfort of the sacred string of beads passing through your fingers will help create a peaceful, restful and restorative space. It may even put you back to sleep.

You might consider creating a special icon, or obtaining one, and placing this in a quiet corner or on a special wall in your home. Russian Orthodox people put a sacred image of the Blessed Mother, Jesus, or another favored saint, in the most visible place in the house, which they call *krasnyi ugol,* the "beautiful corner." Little folding panels with sacred images on them are also set up on an altar for private devotions. Our neighbors in the village always have this little sacred corner or area with pictures of sacred personages and biblical scenes, with candles lit nearby.

These icons, or sacred images, are considered to be holy objects. They speak through an ancient language of imagery and color that inspires serenity and invites meditation. A sacred icon refers to a spiritual dimension and reminds us of the blessed consciousness it portrays. An icon can be an aid to prayer. A precious icon can also be a comfort and be felt as a protection.

Every day you come to pray your rosary will be different. On one day you will feel enthused and inspired, on another, too tired, and on yet another day your mind may be wandering a mile a minute. Some days your prayers will seem especially rich and moving, some days dry and lifeless and at other times somewhere between the two. It is all perfectly fine. Humility, trust and perseverance will serve you well here. Just cross the threshold into the magical grace of the rosary and develop regularity with your recitation, meditating deeply on the mysteries, and you will find your prayer life and your spiritual life blossoming.

Prayer is a living tradition. It includes both spontaneous outpourings of the innermost heart and also implies study, contemplation and a grasp of the spiritual realities one experiences. Our prayers take many forms. The essential forms of all prayer include blessings and adoration, prayers of petition and intercession and prayers of thanksgiving and praise.

Be certain to make an intention for your rosary prayers. Pray for the good of all. Pray for the earth. Pray for peace. Pray for your enemies. Pray for your ancestors. And pray for yourself and those you hold dear. Offer prayers of thanksgiving, as though the things for which you pray are already manifest. And always remember to offer prayers of pure praise, in honor of the Divine spark of life in all things.

"Ask, and it shall be given you; seek and ye shall find; knock and it shall be opened unto you." Matthew 8:7

I truly believe that these prayers of the heart, offered for the benefit of all, will construct a new world order of equality. Fair and equal rights and distribution of the earth's resources, goods and wealth; wholesome food for all; education and health care for all. Concern and protection for the environment, for all living beings and a reversal of modern destructive trends. Peace on earth in our time.

These are the things we want. We can and will bring them about through our collective prayers.

Become a voice actively praying for the earth community...

This does not mean that we do nothing but pray. It means that prayer is essentially the foundation for all we do. And it will naturally lead us in the direction that we need to go.

Every one of us has been called. Through our prayers, we can touch the hearts of all people." Grandmother Agnes

Bring yourself to your rosary, like the old women of my village do, no matter what life has brought to you. Your practice of rosary prayer will become a fountain of spiritual grace, strength and inspiration from which you can continually draw.

The Compendium of the Catechism of the Catholic Church teaches that the fruits of prayer are: charity, joy, peace, patience, kindness, goodness, generosity, gentleness, faithfulness, modesty, self-control and chastity. It lists seven spiritual works of mercy that spring from a vibrant prayer life: to counsel the doubtful, instruct the ignorant, admonish the sinner, comfort the afflicted, forgive offenses, bear wrongs patiently and to pray for the living and the dead. These are the things we are called to do.

"Spirituality's highest purpose is to touch a mystery beyond words, which is perceived only in silence and solitude, the Grandmother's say. Listening within the silence puts one in touch with the energy, vibration, and spiritual forces that are at the heart of Creation. The realms are real, not of the imagination, and can only be reached by a quiet mind and practice." Carol Schaefer, Grandmothers Counsel the World.

The Grandmothers are a group of thirteen indigenous elder women who met in Phoenicia, New York, during October 2004. They came together from the far corners of the world, from such diverse places as the Black Hills of South Dakota, the mountains of Tibet, the jungles of South

America and the rain forest of Africa. Their intention is to form a new global alliance of prayer, education and healing.

"Think always to benefit others and to do no harm."
Tsering Dolma Gyaltong, Grandmother from Tibet

The *Grandmothers* believe that all of our individual ancestral ways of prayer, peacemaking and healing are vitally needed today, and that the teachings of our ancestors will light our way through an unsure future.

They tell us: *"We women have been gifted – we are all-knowing, the creators and makers of life, the seed carriers of the children of the Earth. We must be strong and walk in our innate knowledge and power under the protection of the four directions. With the world on the brink of destruction, women must wake up this great force they possess and bring the world back to peace and harmony. When women and men set in motion this enormously transformative feminine force of unconditional love they carry within, great healing and change will come about."*

The great goal of the *Grandmothers* is to unite the hearts of the world. They agree that self healing is the essential first step toward healing the world. They encourage us to tap into the vast reservoir of vitalizing energy running beneath our common ground and *"centered around a powerful and universal spirituality, based on reverence for our Mother Earth and a shared awareness of the sacredness and interdependence of all life. This creative power of women united is an unmatched force for good."* Carol Schaefer

And in the time honored tradition of wise women through the ages, The *Grandmothers* offer us this prophecy: *"A new consciousness is to be created that will combine the accomplishments of the mind and the deep wisdom of the heart, which is the key to a prosperous and sustainable future for all." Mayan Grandmother Flordemayo*

Traditionally the Joyful Mysteries are said on Monday and Saturday, Luminous Mysteries on Thursday, Sorrowful Mysteries on Tuesday and Friday and Glorious Mysteries on Wednesday and Sunday. But these are merely guidelines. Allow spirit to move you, and meditate on the mysteries that hold a special appeal to your heart on any given day.

Following are the sacred mystery stories of the rosary and the traditional plants, foods and medicines associated with them.

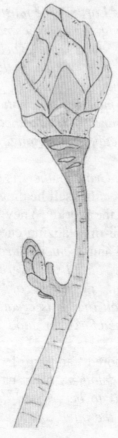

THE MYSTERIES OF THE ROSARY

THE JOYFUL MYSTERIES

The Joyful Mysteries express the joy and exultation of the Incarnation. They bring us excitement, delight, jubilation and anticipation. These are the mysteries of conception. They speak to us of beginnings and of creative becoming.

The Joyful Mysteries remind us that our Christian faith is at its very core, "good news." On the sacred wheel of life, these first five mysteries sit firmly in the east.

Each of the Joyful Mysteries is a paradox. Holding both the light and dark in balance, they emphasize the yin/yang of life present within each situation. They speak to us about stepping fully into each new moment and being truly ourselves.

THE ANNUNCIATION TO MARY

THE VISITATION

THE BIRTH OF JESUS

THE PRESENTATION OF JESUS IN THE TEMPLE

FINDING JESUS IN THE TEMPLE

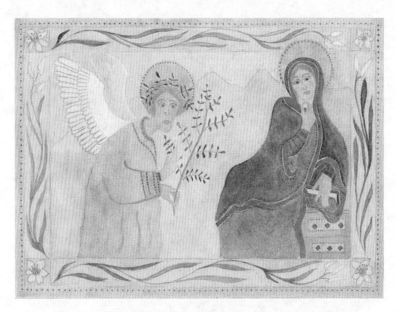

THE ANNUNCIATION TO MARY

The Archangel Gabriel tells the Virgin Mary that she is about to become the Mother of God. Mary accepts, declaring herself to be the "Handmaid of the Lord."

The angel Gabriel was sent by God to a town in Galilee called Nazareth. There he visited a young virgin by the name of Mary who was betrothed to a man named Joseph, of the House of David.

He went in and said to her, "Rejoice, you who enjoy God's favor! The Lord is with you." She was deeply disturbed by these words and asked herself what this greeting could mean.

The angel then said to her, "Mary, do not be afraid; you have won God's favor. Look! You are to conceive in your womb and bear a son, and you will name him Jesus. He will be great and will be called Son of the Most High. The Lord God will give him the throne of his ancestor David;

he will rule over the House of Jacob forever and his reign will have no end."

Mary said to the angel, "But how can this come about since I have no knowledge of man?"

And the angel answered, "The Holy Spirit will come over you, and the power of the Most High will cover you with its shadow. And so the child will be holy and will be called Son of God.

"And I tell you this too: your cousin Elizabeth also, in her old age, has conceived a son, and she whom the people called barren is now in her sixth month, for nothing is impossible to God."

And Mary said, "You see before you the Lord's servant, let it be done to me as you have said. And the angel left her. Luke 1:26-38

Plants associated with the Annunciation – white lily *Lilium candidum,* olive *Olea europea,* violet *Viola odorata,* fuchsia *Fuchsia magellanica*

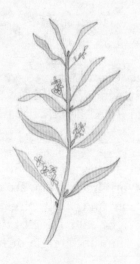

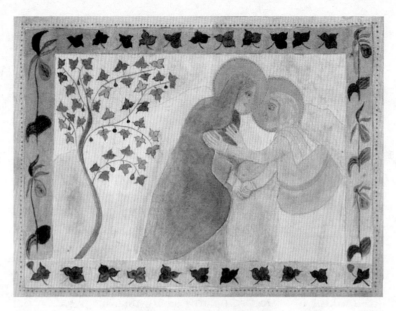

THE VISITATION

Mary sets out to visit St. Elizabeth who was carrying St. John the Baptist in her womb.

Mary immediately set out into the hill country to a town in Judah. She went into Zachariah's house and greeted Elizabeth.

It happened that as soon as Elizabeth heard Mary's greeting, the child leapt in her womb and Elizabeth was filled with the Holy Spirit.

She cried out, "Of all women you are the most blessed, and blessed is the fruit of your womb. Why should I be honored with a visit from the mother of my Lord? Look, the moment your greeting reached my ears, the child in my womb leapt for joy. Yes, blessed is she who believed that the promise made her by the Lord would be fulfilled."

And Mary said: "My soul proclaims the greatness of the Lord and my spirit rejoices in God my Savior; because he has looked upon the humiliation of his servant.

"Yes, from now onwards all generations will call me blessed, for the Almighty has done great things for me. Holy is his name, and his faithful love extends age after age to those who love him.

"He has used the power of his arm; he has routed the arrogant of heart. He has pulled princes down from their thrones and raised high the lowly. He has filled the starving with good things and sent the rich away empty.

"He has come to the help of Israel his servant mindful of his faithful love according to the promise he made to our ancestors."

Mary stayed with her cousin Elizabeth for three months until the baby was born, and then went home. Luke 1:39-55

Plants associated with The Visitation – The fig tree *Ficus carica*, Our Lady's slipper *Cypripedium calceolus*, iris *Iris germanica*, peony *Paeonia officinalis*, and rose, *Rosa spp.*

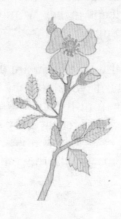

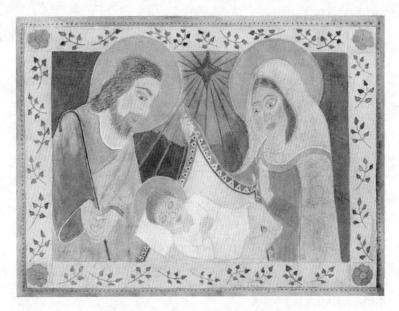

THE BIRTH OF JESUS

Jesus was born in a grotto in Bethlehem.

Now at that time Caesar Augustus issued a decree that a census should be made of the whole inhabited world. This census, the first, took place while Quirinius was governor of Syria, and everyone went to be registered, each to his or her own town.

So Joseph set out from the town of Nazareth in Galilee for Judea, to David's town called Bethlehem, since he was of David's House and line, in order to be registered together with Mary, his betrothed who was with child.

Now it happened that, while they were there, the time came for her to have her child, and she gave birth to a son, her first-born. She wrapped him in swaddling clothes and laid him in a manger because there was no room for them in the living-space.

Nearby in the fields there were shepherds keeping watch over their sheep during the night. An angel of the Lord shone round them. They were terrified, but the angel said, "Do not be afraid. Look, I bring you good news of great joy, a joy to be shared by the whole people. Today in the town of David a Savior has been born to you; he is Christ the Lord. And here is a sign for you: you will find a baby wrapped in swaddling clothes and lying in a manger. And all at once with the angel there was a great throng of the hosts of heaven, praising God with the words: Glory to God in the highest heaven, and on earth peace for all.

Now it happened that when the angels had gone from them into heaven, the shepherds said to one another, "Let us go to Bethlehem and see this event which the Lord has made known to us."

So they hurried away and found Mary and Joseph, and the baby lying in the manger. When they saw the child they repeated what they had been told about him, and everyone who heard it was astonished at what the shepherds said to them.

As for Mary, she treasured all these things and pondered them in her heart. And the shepherds went back glorifying and praising God for all they had heard and seen, just as it had been told. Luke 2:1-20

Plants associated with The Birth of Jesus – Rose *Rosa spp.*, star of Bethlehem *Ornithogalum umbellatum*, Christmas rose *Helleborus niger*, bedstraw *Galium spp.*

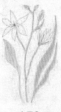

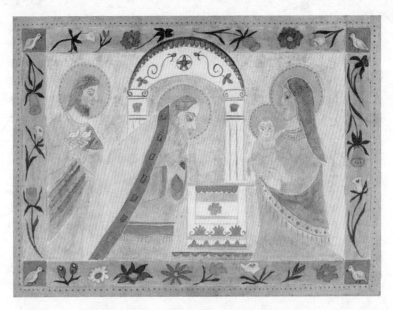

THE PRESENTATION OF JESUS IN THE TEMPLE

Mary and Joseph, faithful to the Law of Moses, present their baby Jesus in the Temple and fulfill that which was prescribed for their purification.

And when the day came for Jesus and Mary to be purified in keeping with the Law of Moses, they took him up to Jerusalem to present him to the Lord – observing what is written in the Law of the Lord – Every first-born male must be consecrated to the Lord. - and also to offer a sacrifice, in accordance with what is prescribed in the Law of the Lord, a pair of turtle doves or two young pigeons.

Now in Jerusalem there was a man named Simeon. He was an upright and devout man: he looked forward to the restoration of Israel, and the Holy Spirit rested on him.

It had been revealed to him by the Holy Spirit that he would not see death until he had set eyes on the Christ of the Lord. Prompted by the Spirit he came to the Temple; and when the parents brought in the child Jesus to do for him what the law required, he took him into his arms and blessed God and said: "Now Master, you are letting your servant go in peace as you promised; for my eyes have seen the salvation which you have made ready in the sight of the nations; a light of revelation for the gentiles and glory for your people Israel."

As the child's father and mother were wondering at the things that were being said about him, Simeon blessed them and said to Mary his mother, "Look, he is destined for the fall and the rise of many in Israel, destined to be a sign that is opposed – and a sword will pierce your heart also – so that the secret prayers of many may be laid bare."

There was a prophetess too, Anna, the daughter of Phanuel, of the tribe of Asher. She was well on in years. Her days of girlhood over, she had been married for seven years before becoming a widow.

She was now eighty-four years old and never left the Temple, serving God night and day with fasting and prayer. She came up just at that moment and began to praise God, and she spoke of the child to all who looked forward to the deliverance of Jerusalem. Luke 2:22-38

Plants associated with The Presentation – all spring herbs and flowers, especially crocus *Crocus vernus*, snowdrops *Galanthus nivallis*, hyacinth *Hyacinthus orientalis* and daffodil *Narcissus psuedonarc*.

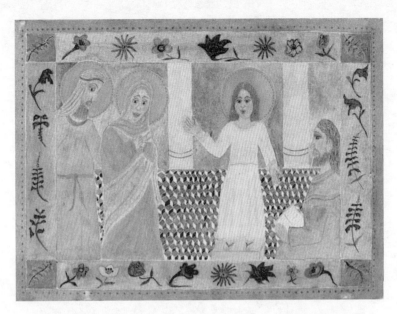

FINDING JESUS IN THE TEMPLE

The child Jesus remained for three days in the Temple in Jerusalem, unknown to Mary and Joseph.

Every year Jesus' parents went to Jerusalem for the feast of the Passover. When he was twelve years old, they went up for the feast as usual.

When the days of the feast were over and they set off for home, the boy Jesus stayed behind in Jerusalem without his parents knowing it. They assumed he was somewhere in the party, and it was only after a day's journey that they went to look for him among their relations and acquaintances. When they failed to find him, they went back to Jerusalem looking for him everywhere.

It happened that, three days later, they found him in the Temple, sitting among the teachers, listening to them, and asking them questions, and all those who heard him were astounded at his intelligence and his replies.

Mary and Joseph were overcome when they saw him and his mother said to him, "My child, why have you done this to us? See how worried your father and I have been, looking for you."

He replied, "Why were you looking for me? Did you not know that I must be in my Father's house?" But they did not understand what he meant.

He went down with them and came to Nazareth and lived under their authority.

His mother stored up all these things in her heart. And Jesus increased in wisdom, in stature, and in favor with God and with people. Luke 2:41-52

Plants associated with Finding Jesus in the Temple - anemone *Anemone nemerosa*, obedient plant *Psychostegia virginiana,* and the spring blossoming herbs and flowers of field and wood.

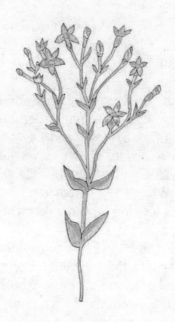

THE LUMINOUS MYSTERIES

The Luminous Mysteries, or mysteries of light, describe the public life of Jesus as he reveals himself as *The Light of the World*. These are the mysteries of doing and of being. These mysteries bring our awareness to our responsibility toward humanity, encouraging us to act with humility and kindness. They beckon us to follow the calling of our hearts, to follow our dreams. As mysteries that epitomize our work in the world, the Luminous Mysteries are clearly positioned at the southern quadrant of the sacred wheel of life.

The Luminous Mysteries exemplify the mission of Christ and his nourishing, redemptive gifts, and meditating on these mysteries sheds light on our own personal mission in the world and the contributions we have to offer as well.

Though Mary is mostly in the background of these mysteries, her presence with Jesus is strongly felt. Her words at the wedding in Cana, "Do whatever he tells you," resound through these mystery stories and reverberate across the ages.

THE BAPTISM OF JESUS IN THE JORDAN

JESUS CHANGES WATER TO WINE AT CANA

JESUS PROCLAIMS THE KINGDOM OF GOD AND FORGIVES SINS

JESUS TRANSFIGURED ON MOUNT TABOR

JESUS OFFERS US THE EUCHARIST

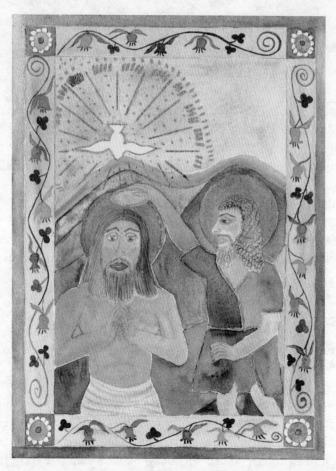

THE BAPTISM OF JESUS

Jesus is baptized by John the Baptist in the Jordan River.

It was at this time that Jesus came from Nazareth in Galilee and was baptized in the Jordan by John. And at once, as he was coming out of the water, he saw the heavens torn apart and the Spirit, like a dove, descending on him. And a voice came from heaven, "You are my Son, the Beloved; my favor rests on you." Mark 1:9

Plants associated with The Baptism of Jesus – Columbine *Aquilegia vulgaris*.

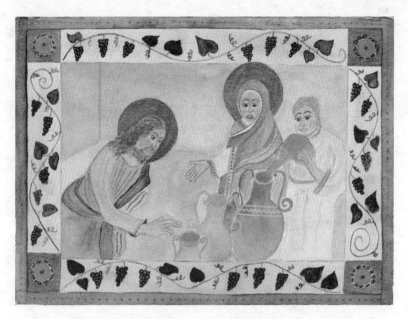

JESUS CHANGES WATER INTO WINE AT THE WEDDING IN CANA

The first of the signs took place at Cana when, due to the intervention of Mary, Jesus changed water into wine.

They ran out of wine…and the mother of Jesus said to him, "They have no wine."

Jesus said: "Woman, what do you want from me? My hour has not yet come."

And his mother said to the servants: "Do whatever he tells you." John 2:3-5

Plants associated with Changing Water into Wine - Grapes *Vitis vinifera*.

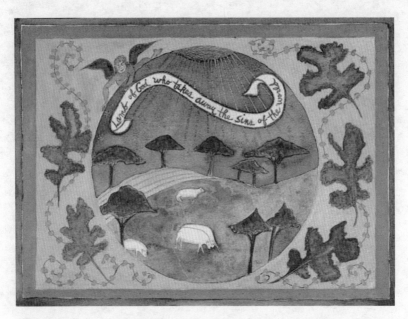

JESUS PROCLAIMS THE KINGDOM OF GOD AND THE FORGIVENESS OF SINS

By preaching, healing and miracles Jesus proclaims the Kingdom of God, calls all who can hear, and forgives the sins of those who draw near to him in humble trust.

And Jesus went about all the cities and villages, teaching in their synagogues, and preaching the gospel of the kingdom, and healing every sickness and every disease among the people. Matthew 9:35-36

After John was arrested, Jesus went into Galilee. There he proclaimed the gospel of God, saying,"The time is fulfilled, and the kingdom of God is close at hand. Repent, and believe in the Gospel." Mark 1:14-15

Plants associated with Jesus Proclaiming the Kingdom of God and Forgiving Sins – Mustard family plants, the *Brassicas*.

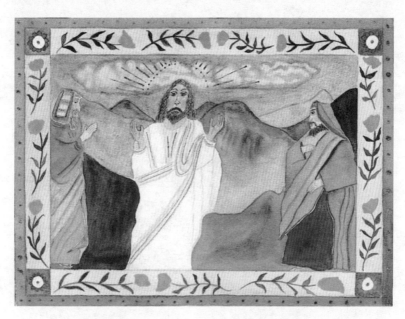

JESUS IS TRANSFIGURED ON MOUNT TABOR

Jesus takes three disciples with him to the top of a high mountain and he is transfigured before them.

And it came to pass that Jesus took Peter, John and James and went up on the mountain to pray. And as he prayed, the fashion of his countenance was altered, and his raiment was white and glistening.

And behold, there talked with him two men, which were Moses and Elias...A cloud came and covered them with a shadow…and a voice came from the cloud saying, "This is my Beloved Son, hear him." Luke 9:28-29, 34-35

Plants associated with Jesus Transfigured on Mount Tabor – Goldenrod *Solidago spp*, almond tree *Prunus amaygdalus*

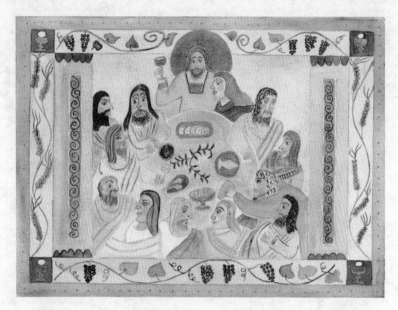

JESUS OFFERS US THE EUCHARIST

Christ institutes the Eucharist at the Last Supper, offering his body and blood and asking us to do this in remembrance of him.

Now as they were eating, Jesus took bread, and blessed and broke it, and gave it to his disciples and said, "Take, eat; this is my body." And he took a cup and when he had given thanks he gave it to them, saying, "Drink of it, all of you; for this is my blood of the covenant, which is poured out for many for the forgiveness of sins."...

And when they had sung a hymn, they went out into the Mount of Olives.

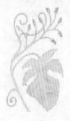 **Plants associated with The Gift of the Eucharist** – grapes *Vitis vinifera*, and wheat *Triticum aestivum*.

THE SORROWFUL MYSTERIES

The abject suffering of the Sorrowful Mysteries is heartbreaking. These mysteries reveal the depths of love, faith and commitment and speak about the power of transformation. They bring our awareness to the ultimate death and dissolution of all living things. Because the Sorrowful Mysteries cause us to feel such deep and painful emotion, they are firmly situated in the western section of the sacred wheel of life.

We walk with Mary, who walks alongside Jesus on the way to Golgotha. Standing at the foot of the cross with Mary, we become one with her agony, despair and desolation. She is the Dark of the Moon, the Sorrowful Mother, standing at the edge of the world, at the edge of all time. Her beloved son, the Son of God, is dead. This is the nadir of the mysteries, the lowest point.

> You are the moon and the tides
> and the mysteries of birth and death
> you are the star shine
> and passion's witness
> you show us the way
> through the portal of despair
> into wholeness.

THE AGONY IN THE GARDEN OF GETHSEMANE

THE SCOURGING AT THE PILLAR

THE CROWNING WITH THORNS

THE CARRYING OF THE CROSS

THE CRUCIFIXION AND DEATH OF JESUS

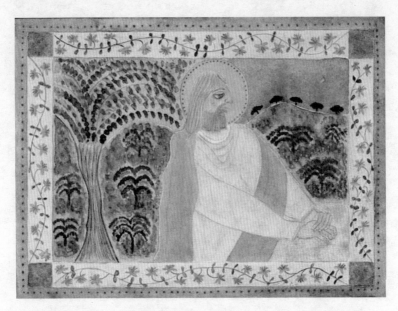

THE AGONY IN THE GARDEN OF GETHSEMANE

Before his passion, Jesus prayed that the suffering and death he faced might be taken away, but also willed to fulfill whatever the Father wanted of him.

Now Jesus and his disciples came to a plot of land called Gethsemane, and he said to his disciples, "Stay here while I pray."

Then he took Peter and James and John with him. And he began to feel terror and anguish. And he said to them, "My soul is sorrowful to the point of death. Wait here, and stay awake."

And going on a little farther he threw himself on the ground and prayed that, if it were possible, this hour might pass him by. "Abba, Father!" he said, "For you everything is possible. Take this cup from me. But let it be as you, not I, would have it."

He came back and found them sleeping, and he said to Peter, "Simon, are you asleep? Had you not the strength to stay awake one hour? Stay awake and pray not to be put to the test. The spirit is willing enough, but human nature is weak."

Again he went away and prayed, saying the same words. And once more he came back and found them sleeping, their eyes were so heavy; and they could find no answer for him.

He came back a third time and said to them, "You can sleep on now and have your rest. It is all over. The hour has come. Now the Son of man is to be betrayed into the hands of sinners.

Get up! Let us go! My betrayer is not far away. Mark 14:32-42

Plants associated with Jesus Praying at the Garden of Gethsemane – Olive *Olea europea*, iris *Iris germanica*, and St. John's wort *Hypericum perforatum*.

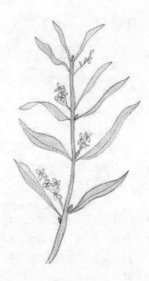

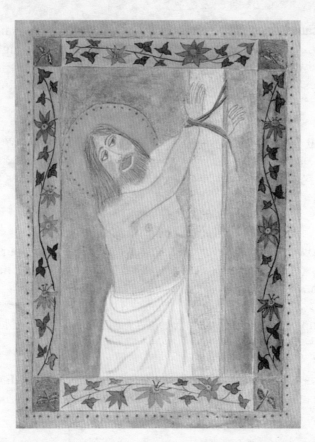

THE SCOURGING AT THE PILLAR

At the hands of the tribunal, Jesus endured a cruel and bloody scourging.

Then Pilate went out again to the Jews and said, "I find no case against him. Would you like me, then, to release for you the king of the Jews?" At this they shouted: "Not this man, but Barabbas"…Pilate then had Jesus taken away and scourged." John 18:38-40, 19:1.

Plants associated with The Scourging at the Pillar – Yarrow *Achillea millefolium,* Knotweed *Polygonum persicaria,* St. John's wort *Hypericum perforatum,* Passion flower *Passiflora incarnata.*

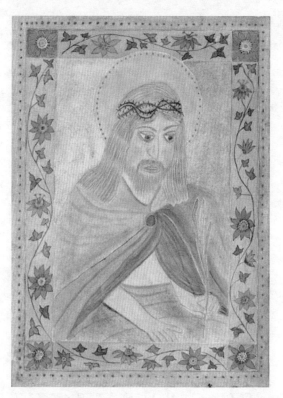

JESUS IS CROWNED WITH THORNS

A crown of thorns was placed on his head.

The soldiers took Jesus with them into the Praetorium and collected the whole battalion around him. And they stripped him and put a scarlet cloak round him, and having plaited thorns into a crown they put this on his head and placed a reed in his right hand. To mock him they knelt to him saying, "Hail, king of the Jews!" And they spat on him and took the reed and struck him on the head with it. Then they led him away to be crucified.

Plants associated with Crowning Jesus with Thorns Crown of thorns *Euphorbia splendens*, St. John's wort *Hypericum perforatum*, passionflower *Passiflora incarnata*.

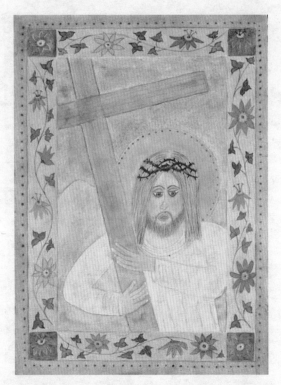

JESUS CARRIES THE CROSS

Condemned to death, Jesus is forced to carry the heavy weight of the cross on his shoulders.

As they led Jesus away, they seized on a man, Simon from Cyrene, coming from the country, and made him shoulder the cross and carry it behind Jesus.

Many of the people walked alongside him, and women too, who mourned and lamented for him. But Jesus turned to them and said, "Daughters of Jerusalem, do not weep for me; weep rather for yourselves and for your children…" Luke 23: 26-29

Plants associated with Jesus Carrying the Cross – Yarrow *Achillea millefolium*, Passion flower *Passiflora incarnata*, St. John's wort *Hypericum perforatum*.

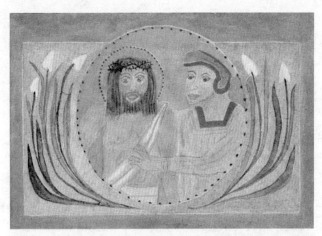

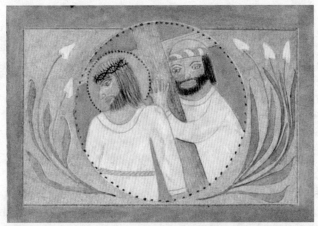

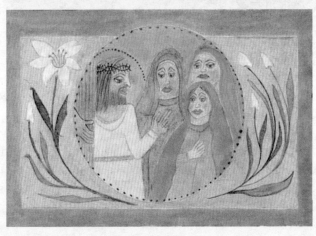

The soldiers offered Jesus wine mixed with myrrh, but he refused it. Then they crucified him, and shared out his clothing, casting lots to decide what each should get. It was the third hour when they crucified him.

The inscription giving the charge against him read, "The King of the Jews." And they crucified two bandits with him, one on the right side and one on the left.

Passersby jeered at him; they shook their heads and said, "So you would destroy the Temple and rebuilt it in three days! Then save yourself; come down from the cross!"

The chief priests and the scribes mocked him among themselves in the same way with the words, "He saved others, he cannot save himself. Let the Christ, the king of Israel, come down from the cross now, for us to see it and believe." Even those who were crucified with him taunted him.

When the sixth hour came, there was darkness over the whole land until the ninth hour. And at the ninth hour Jesus cried out in a loud voice, *"Eloi, eloi, lama sabachthani?"* which means, "My God, my God, why have you forsaken me?"

When some of those who stood nearby heard this, they said, "Listen, he is calling on Elijah." Someone ran and soaked a sponge in vinegar and, putting it on a reed, gave it to him to drink, saying, "Wait! And see if Elijah will come to take him down."

But Jesus gave a loud cry and breathed his last. And the veil of the Sanctuary was torn in two from top to bottom. The centurion, who was standing in front of him, had seen how he died, and he said, "In truth this man was the Son of God."

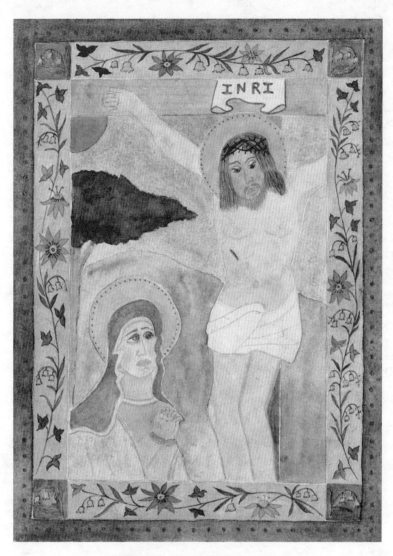

THE CRUCIFIXION AND DEATH OF JESUS

Stripped of his clothes and nailed to the cross, Jesus dies in agony, forgiving his enemies and surrendering his spirit. His last concern was the care of his mother Mary.

There were some women watching from a distance...These used to follow him and look after him when he was in Galilee. And many other women were there who had come up to Jerusalem with him. Mark 15:23-41

Near the foot of the cross of Jesus stood his mother and his mother's sister, Mary the wife of Clopas, and Mary of Magdala. Seeing his mother and the disciple whom he loved standing near her, Jesus said to his mother, "Woman, this is your son."

Then to the disciple he said, "This is your mother." And from that hour the disciple took her into *his* home. John 19:26-28

Plants associated with The Crucifixion and Death of Jesus - Passionflower *Passiflora incarnata*, St. John's wort *Hypericum perforatum*, Maidenhair Fern (Mary's Tears) *Adiantum capillis veneris,* Aloe, *Aloe vera.*

THE GLORIOUS MYSTERIES

The Glorious mysteries bring us full circle. They enrapture us. They free us from fixed thinking and present us with the mystery of faith, essential for living life wholesomely, reverently.

The Glorious mysteries speak to us about life and about the joy inherent in living. They are a celebration! Jesus and Mary show us in a lush and emotional poetry of word, action and imagery about life after death, about the circle of all things, about transformation, rebirth and renewal. Since on the sacred wheel of life the north represents these very aspects, the Glorious Mysteries are situated magnificently in the northern quadrant.

The Glorious mystery stories are mysteries of hope and of rewards richly deserved and rightly granted. We experience the indescribable joy of Mary; her son lives! And she is crowned with his glory. Queen of the Angels, Queen of the Saints. Queen of Heaven and Earth.

We realize our true place, gathered around Mary. We, her people, are the real and timeless face of the church.

THE RESURRECTION

JESUS ASCENDS TO HEAVEN

THE DESCENT OF THE HOLY SPIRIT

THE ASSUMPTION OF THE BLESSED VIRGIN

MARY IS CROWNED QUEEN OF HEAVEN

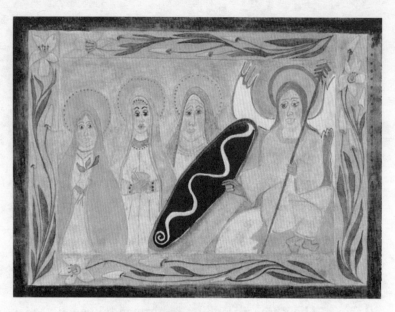

THE RESURRECTION OF JESUS

On the third day Jesus rose from the grave and appeared to many of the disciples over the next forty days.

When the Sabbath was over, Mary of Magdala, Mary the mother of James, and Salome brought spices with which to go and anoint him. And very early in the morning on the first day of the week they went to the tomb when the sun had risen.

They had been saying to one another, "Who will roll away the stone for us from the entrance to the tomb?" But when they looked they saw that the stone, which was very big, had already been rolled back.

On entering the tomb they saw a young man in a white robe seated on the right-hand side, and they were struck with amazement. But he said to them, "There is no need to be amazed. You are looking for Jesus of Nazareth, who was crucified; he has risen, he is not here." Mark 16: 1-8

Mary was stranding outside the tomb weeping. (The angel said) "Woman, why are you weeping?" "They have taken my Lord away," she replied, "and I don't know where they have put him." As she said this she turned around and saw Jesus.

Jesus said to her, "Woman, why are you weeping? Who are you looking for?" Supposing him to be the gardener, she said, "Sir, if you have taken him away, tell me where you have put him and I will go and remove him." Jesus said, "Mary!" She turned around then and said to him in Hebrew, "*Rabbuni!*" which means teacher.

Jesus said to her, "Do not cling to me, because I have not yet ascended to the Father. But go to the others and tell them: I am ascending to my Father and your Father, to my God and your God."

So Mary of Magdala told the disciples, "I have seen the Lord," and that he had said these things to her. John 20:10-18

Plants associated with The Resurrection – Easter lily *Lilium longiflora,* resurrection plant *Anastatica hierochuntica*, pomegranate *Punica granatum*, spikenard *Nardostachys jatamansi*, lily of the valley *Convallaria majellis*, myrrh *Commiphora gileadensis*, *Aloe vera*, saffron *Crocus sativus*, palm *Phoenix dactylifera*, cypress *Cupressus sempervirens*, chicory *Cichorlum intybus.*

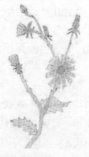

JESUS ASCENDS TO HEAVEN

The risen Lord ascended into heaven where he sits in glory awaiting his return at the end of time.

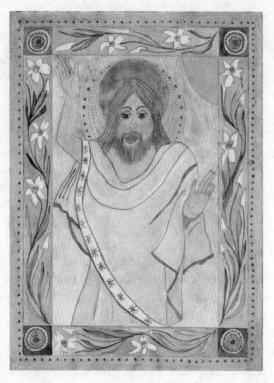

Then Jesus took the disciples out to the outskirts of Bethany (to the Mount of Olives) and then raising up his hands he blessed them. Now as he blessed them, he withdrew from them and was carried up to heaven. They worshiped him and then went back to Jerusalem full of joy; and they were continually in the Temple praising God. Luke 24: 50-53

While they were standing there looking intently at the sky as he was leaving, suddenly two men dressed in white garments stood beside them and said, "Men of Galilee, why are you standing here gazing at the sky? This Jesus who has been taken up from you into heaven will return one day in the same way as you have seen him going up to heaven." Acts 1:9-11

Plants associated with The Ascension of Jesus into Heaven – Jacobs ladder *Polemonium caerul*, Easter lily *Lilium longiflora*, chicory *Cichorlum intybus*.

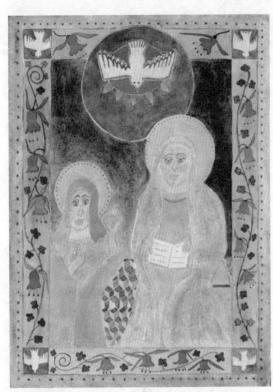

THE DESCENT OF THE HOLY SPIRIT

As Jesus promised, the Holy Spirit descended upon Mary and the disciples on the Feast of Pentecost, strengthening and enlightening them.

When the days of Pentecost were drawing to a close they were all gathered together in the same place. All of a sudden there came from the sky a rumbling like that of a strong driving wind, filling the whole house where they were assembled.

Tongues as of fire appeared which parted and came to rest on each of them. They were filled with the Holy Spirit and began to express themselves in other tongues as Holy Spirit enabled them to speak. Acts 2:1-4

I shall pour out my spirit on all people. Your sons and daughters shall prophecy, your young people shall see visions, and your old people dream dreams. Acts 2:17-18

Plants associated with The Descent of the Holy Spirit – red columbine *Aquilegia canadensis*, pinks *Dianthus plumarius*, philodendron *Philodendron wilsonii*.

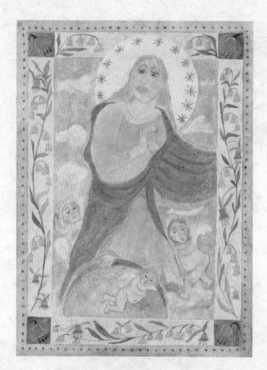

THE ASSUMPTION OF MARY INTO HEAVEN

At the end of her life, Mary was assumed body and soul into heaven where she reigns in glory with her Son.

Then a great sign appeared in the sky, a woman clothed with the sun, with the moon under her feet and a crown of twelve stars on her head. Revelation 12:1

My love lifts up his voice, he says to me, "Come then, my beloved, my lovely one, come. For see, winter is past, the rains are over and gone. Flowers are appearing on the earth. The season of glad songs has come." Song of Songs 2:10-13

Plants associated with the Assumption - Assumption lily *Hosta plantaginia*, lily of the valley *Convallaria majellis*, pomegranate *Punica granatum*, myrrh *Commiphora gileadensis*, spikenard *Nardostachys jatamansi*

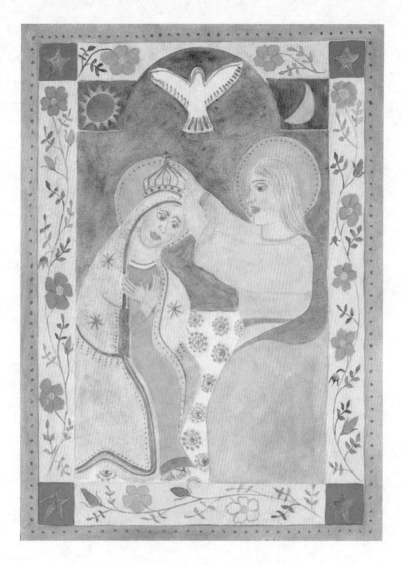

CORONATION OF MARY AS QUEEN OF HEAVEN

Mary is crowned Queen of Heaven and is seated in glory among the angels and saints of heaven. She is the first fruit of redeemed humanity.

And Mary said: My soul proclaims the greatness of the Lord and my spirit rejoices in God my Savior; because he has looked upon the humiliation of his servant. Yes, from now onwards all generations will call me blessed, for the Almighty has done great things for me. Holy is his name" Luke 1:46-49

Plants associated with The Coronation of Mary – roses and all *Rosacea* family plants.

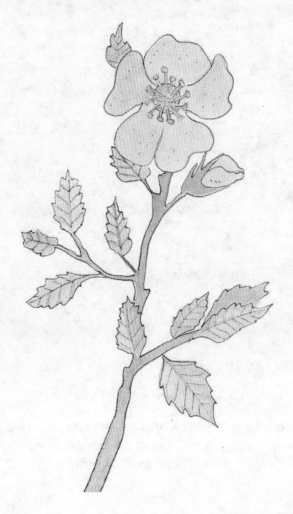

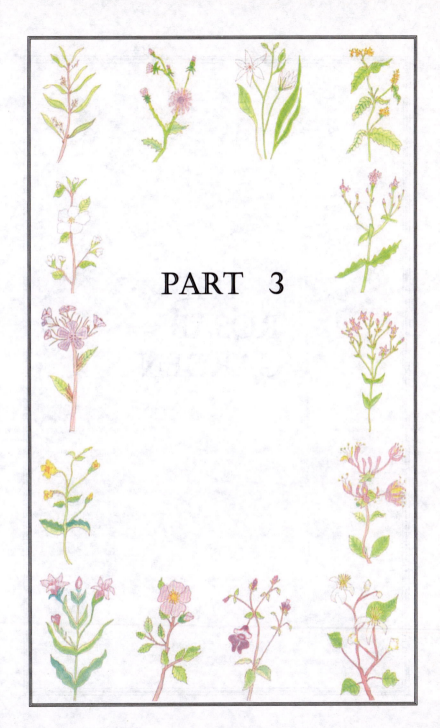

PART 3

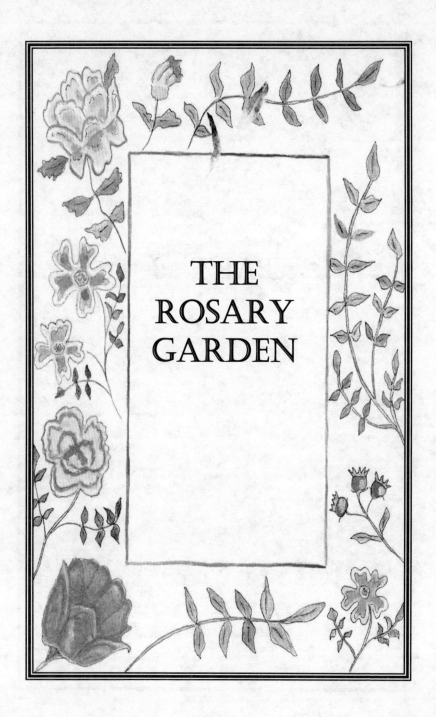

THE ROSARY GARDEN

The rosary mysteries focus our minds and hearts on the story of our birth as a people, as a culture. They also speak to us of certain plants, herbs and foods of field and wood, necessary for our sustenance. These plants became associated with each of the mysteries and their teachings due to their individual features and unique qualities. These included the growing habit; the color, form and aroma of the flowers, leaves and in some cases, roots; its natural habitat; and the over-all effect of its use on other living beings, such as its specific medicinal, spiritual and emotional benefits.

The JOYFUL MYSTERIES bring our attention to the Allium and Liliaceae Family plants (Lily, garlic, onions etc.), Figs, and the spring and summer herbs and flowers of field and garden (Mary's Florilegia or Mary's flowers).

The LUMINOUS MYSTERIES concentrate on Grapes and fermented food and drink, Brassica Family plants (broccoli, mustard, radish, etc.) and the Cereals, such as wheat, oats, barley and rye.

The SORROWFUL MYSTERIES highlight The Olive Tree, St. John's wort, Aloe Vera and Passion flower.

The GLORIOUS MYSTERIES celebrate Mary's Emblem, the Mystical Rose and the nourishing Rosaceae Family plants, such as hawthorn, apple, raspberry and strawberry.

All of these plants and foods together present us with an excellent all-around foundation for good health.

Welcome to my Rosary Garden. Come walk along these mystical garden paths with me as we rediscover heirloom truths long hidden deep within the stories these particular plants have to t

OUR LADY'S FLORILEGIA

TEACHINGS OF THE HERBS FLOWERS AND TREES OF THE MYSTERIES

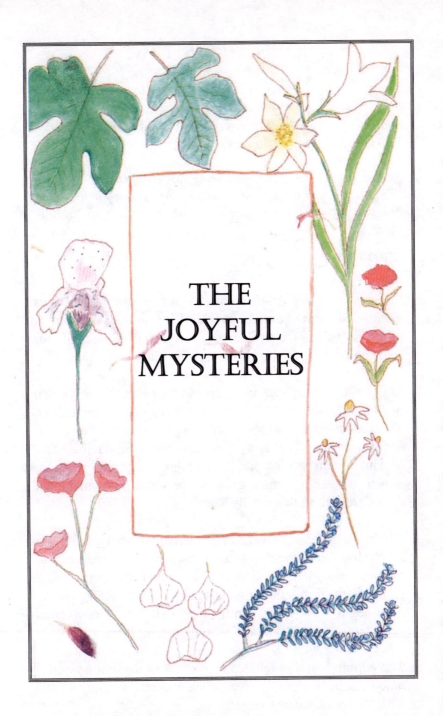

THE JOYFUL MYSTERIES

JOYFUL MYSTERIES

In the Joyful Mysteries we will focus on the edible Alliums and Liliaceae Family plants (Lily, garlic, onions etc.), Figs and the herbs and flowers of field and garden (Mary's Florilegia or Mary's flowers).

In days of old, the Alliaceae Family was considered part of the Liliaceae Family but has now been given its own family status. For our purposes we will include both plant families together here.

THE ALLIUM AND LILIACEAE FAMILY

Liliaceae is a large plant family with at least 3,500 species distributed throughout the world. They include hyacinths, tulips, as well as the true lilies. These are all flowers of Our Lady and can easily be grown in your Mary garden.

Many native members of Liliaceae make excellent garden plants, such as the Alliums, Brodiaea, Camassia, Lilium and Calochortus species, which prefer to grow in open, sunny areas. Trillium, Erythronium, Smilacina and Maianthemum prefer shaded habitats and require more moisture over a longer growing period. The medicinal Aloes are also in this family.

All species of Liliaceae are perennial, but most are herbaceous and die back after flowering or fruiting, to survive as underground bulbs, corms or rhizomes. New plants form from bulb division or sprout from seeds, but do not begin flowering until the bulb has developed sufficiently, which can take as long as four years.

The Allium Family includes vegetables of the onion family: onion, garlic, leek and chives. The majority are herbaceous with a swollen storage organ.

CHARACTERISTICS:

Bulbs or other storage organs; long, thin leaves; six flower petals; six stamens; a seed capsule, which forms inside the flower.

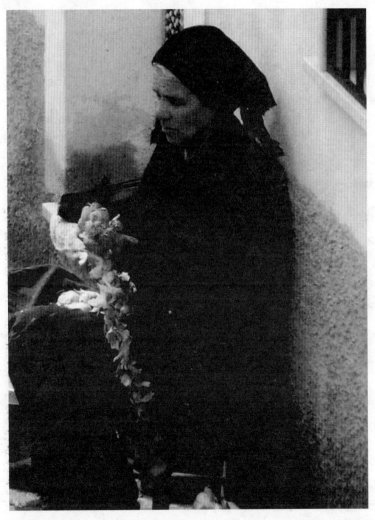

The little fruit and vegetable store in our village has large, beautiful braids of garlic bulbs hanging from the walls. They smell so fresh and wonderful, blending with the vibrant colors and aromas of all the other beautifully displayed foods to make a visit there a high point of almost any day. The oranges all have fresh leaves on them and look and smell like they were just harvested that morning. The eggplants are plump and big. The fleshy black and green olives floating in a heavenly brine are absolutely irresistible. Everything is organically grown and of amazing quality! And it's not just being in the store that makes a visit there so special. It is also the experience of walking there and back. Of course, one has to go before 1:30 or after 4:30 or the store will be closed. Most of the residents of our village take a siesta after their midday meal. Afternoons find the San Giacomese either eating a big happy dinner with their extended family and neighbors or in repose until the late afternoon church bells ring.

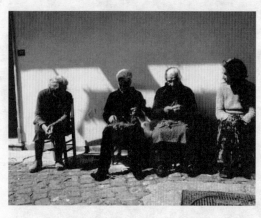

The women often sit outside their houses on tiny wooden chairs set in a sunny spot and do their work with foods, like braiding garlic or cleaning and trimming freshly gathered greens. I usually stop and sit with them while they work and often lend a hand. I enjoy the laughing and joking that the women do together. I feel happy when they welcome me affectionately by pinching my cheek and kissing me on both sides of my face. And I especially appreciate their generosity when they show up at my door unexpectedly with a plateful of freshly made zepoli, a nice bottle of homemade wine, a block of cheese, or a few bulbs of the wonderful garlic that they grow!

ALLIUM FAMILY The biting aroma of the Allium family plants is due to their sulfur-rich, volatile oil, allicin. This substance is primarily responsible for the power of garlic and onions to kill bacteria and stimulate circulation. There are over 600 species of Alliums, distributed all over Europe, North America, Northern Africa and Asia. The plants are used as ornamentals, vegetables, spices, and as medicine.

The edible Alliums contain iron, are a rich source of vitamins and minerals, and offer a host of other health promoting properties. They are an indispensable addition to the daily diet and their use goes back to at least 3,000 B.C. when they were offered by the Egyptians to their gods.

  Our Lady's Garleek, chives, *Allium schoenoprasum*

  Mary's Garlic, Ramsons, *Allium ursinum*

  The Virgin's Tears, onion, *Allium roseum, A. cepa*

GARLIC - *Allium sativum* was surely one of the earliest spices used to liven up the taste of food.

Garlic is antibacterial, antiviral, antiseptic, antiparasitic, immune-stimulating, antispasmodic, hypotensive (lowers blood pressure), diaphoretic (promotes sweating), antiprotozoan, antifungal and cholagogue (stimulates the flow of bile).

Sumerian cuneiform tablets written in 2,600 B.C. describe the dietary staples of the time and include garlic along with grains, legumes, some root vegetables, leafy greens like lettuce and mustard, cucumbers and a variety of fish.

The Sumerians also recorded using garlic for healing in the medical texts of King Ashurbanipal's library dating 688 to 826 B.C.

Pliny, the Roman naturalist, thought garlic was good for almost every known affliction. Hippocrates, called the Father of Medicine, recommended garlic for infections, wounds, cancer, leprosy and digestive disorders. Dioscorides, chief physician for Nero's army, used it for treating heart problems and as a remedy for coughs and colds, to expel intestinal worms, clear the arteries, eradicate skin rashes, and stimulate hair growth. Galen, the Greek physician, simply called garlic a "cure-all."

Ancient Romans and Greeks considered garlic a symbol of strength and courage, and their athletes, workers and soldiers consumed it regularly. Greek midwives hung garlic cloves in birthing rooms to keep evil spirits away, and this custom became commonplace down through the centuries in most European homes.

The Egyptians held garlic in high esteem and recorded over two hundred medicinal uses for it. Garlic depictions have been found on Egyptian tombs dating back to 3200 B.C. The ancient Hebrews considered garlic to enhance virility and said that "it keeps the body warm, brightens the face, increases semen, kills parasites, fosters love and removes jealousy." The Israelites were so fond of garlic they referred to themselves as "garlic eaters." They relied on the regular use of garlic to keep their bodies functioning optimally, and we can too.

Garlic will help keep the heart healthy, help keep blood pressure down, as well help keep cholesterol levels in check. Chop some into your salad, as my mother always did, or throw it, simmered in olive oil, over noodles and sprinkle with parsley. Paula Wolfert, an expert on Mediterranean cuisine, thinks a mixture of garlic and olive oil is one of the greatest discoveries in culinary history. She says, "When garlic and olive oil are combined in a creamy suspension, something sublime is born."

Jean English, a Maine organic gardener and whole foods aficionado, warns that a mix of garlic and olive oil should be used immediately, or there is a chance that spores of botulism can form.

Garlic is rich in antibiotic powers and is strengthening to the immune system. It is active against both gram positive and gram negative bacteria, including *Shigella dysenteriae, Staphylococcus aureus, Pseudomonas aeruginosa, Candida albicans, Escherichia coli, Streptococcus spp., Salmonella spp., Campylobacter., Proteus mirablis and Bacillus anthracis*. During World War 1, the Russian army used garlic to treat wounds incurred by soldiers on the Front Line. In fact, the Red Army physicians relied so heavily on garlic that it became known as "Russian Penicillin."

Garlic helps fight against herpes simplex, influenza B, HIV and many other serious illnesses. Garlic kills bacteria in the gastrointestinal tract immediately on contact.

Antioxidant garlic is a benefit to those dealing with cancer. Dr. Richard Rivlin of the Sloan-Kettering Institute makes a case for eating a couple of cloves each day to reduce your risk of developing cancer. The American Institute for Cancer Research agrees, adding that garlic may be especially effective for warding off cancer of the esophagus. And research by Dr. John Milner at Penn State indicates that consuming garlic leads to a lower risk of colon cancer.

Garlic stimulates the brain. Eleanor Roosevelt is said to have eaten three chocolate-covered cloves of garlic every day to help keep her memory sharp. And because it helps to increase insulin production, garlic in the diet is helpful in the control of diabetes. Garlic is used to season the foods of almost every culture in the world. Add it to salads, soups, stews, sauces, rice, noodles, vegetable dishes, pickles, fish, poultry, and meats.

On Christmas Eve Italian Catholics traditionally enjoy a meal of fish and pasta. My grandmother always prepared a spaghetti dish covered with garlic simmered in olive oil with a bit of parsley on this special night. We call this dish *Aglio e Olio* My mother made this same dish every Christmas Eve, and now I serve it to my family. I have no doubt that my kids will all prepare *Aglio e Olio* for their families when the time comes. Of course, there is no need to wait until Christmas to enjoy this delightful dish. It is simple and easy to prepare and eat all year round.

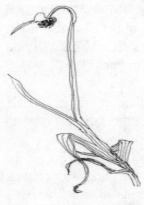

Growing garlic is easy. You can grow a winter's supply in a 3 x 5 bed. The soil needs to be fertile, so add some nourishing compost to ensure a good harvest. We usually plant our garlic around mid-October, but I have also planted garlic bulbs early in spring, as soon as the ground could be worked, and they grew perfectly fine, though perhaps not quite as big.

Fall planted garlic bulbs are among the very first of the spring greens to emerge. Called green garlic, these leaves are a bit thicker than chives and can be eaten cooked or raw. These young garlic greens make a very welcome, enlivening and nourishing addition to any salad. They taste tender and sweet and are a wonderful spring tonic. During the growing season garlic must be kept well weeded, and appreciates watering during dry spells.

We grow garlic on our farm in Maine and can usually expect to harvest it in mid-to late July. When about half of the leaves are drooping and turn brown, it's time to dig. After you've taken the bulbs up from the ground, being careful not to hurt them as you do so, tie six or so in a bunch and hang them in a dry place to cure for a couple of weeks. We usually set aside the biggest ones for the next planting, and eat, store or sell, the rest.

Garlic bulbs have a long shelf life. The soft neck varieties last for nine months or so, the hard necks not quite as long.

ONION – *Allium cepa* – Onions are highly valued both for their culinary as well as their medicinal benefits.

Many archaeologists, botanists and food historians believe onions originated in central Asia. Other research suggests that onions were first grown in Iran and West Pakistan. What we know for certain is that people started eating wild onions very early - long before farming was invented. This humble wild vegetable was no doubt a staple food in the prehistoric diet.

The Egyptians cultivated onions for at least six thousand years and recorded the importance of onions as a food as well as its use in art, religion, medicine and mummification. Onions were regarded by them as a cure-all, considered to possess aphrodisiac properties, and to be a necessity of the daily diet.

In Egypt, onions were an object of worship. The ancient Egyptians conceived of the world as an onion, with the spheres of heaven, earth and hell formed concentrically and in layers, like the onion bulb. The bulb symbolized eternity, and onions were buried alongside the Pharaohs.

Paintings of onions appear on the inner walls of the pyramids and in the tombs and were shown upon the altars of the gods. Frequently, a priest is pictured holding onions in his hand or covering an altar with a bundle of their leaves or bulbs.

Onions have frequently been found packed into the pelvic regions of mummies and also in the thorax, flattened against the ears and in front of the collapsed eyes. Flowering onions have been found on the chest, and onions have been found attached to the soles of the feet and along the legs. King Ramses IV, who died in 1160 B.C., was entombed with onions in his eye sockets.

Onions grew in Chinese gardens as early as 5,000 years ago, and they are referenced in some of the oldest Vedic writings from India. The *Charaka – Sanhita*, a medical text written in the early sixth century B.C., celebrates the onion as a medicine and describes it as being diuretic, good for digestion, the heart, eyes and joints.

A staple of the ancient Hebrew diet was the onion board, consisting of bread dough covered with sautéed onions and poppy seeds and then baked. In Numbers 11:5, the children of Israel lament the meager desert diet enforced by the Exodus: "We remember the fish, which we did eat in Egypt freely, the cucumbers and the melons and the leeks and the onions and the garlic." The Allium family provided a large part of the basis for their daily diet.

The Romans were also fans of onions. Pliny the Elder wrote of Pompeii's magnificent onions and cabbages. He catalogued the Roman beliefs that the onion could cure vision, induce sleep, heal mouth sores and dog bites, toothaches, dysentery and lumbago. Excavators of Pompeii, located south of Naples, found gardens where, just as Pliny said, onions had grown. The bulbs evidently left behind cavities in the ground.

By the Middle Ages, beans, cabbage and onions were the staple vegetables of European cuisine. Onions served not only as a food for the poor and the wealthy alike, but were also prescribed as medicine to alleviate headaches, cure snakebites and prevent hair loss. Bunches of onions were used as rent payment and also presented as wedding gifts.

During the plague people in Medieval Europe hung bunches of onions outside their doors to protect their household against the disease. Syrup made from boiled onions and mixed with honey was used against colds and coughs, and sautéed or boiled onions were placed between two sheets of flannel and placed on the chest to aid pulmonary distress and help bring up phlegm.

The first Pilgrims brought onions with them on the Mayflower but soon found that strains of wild onions already grew throughout the new land. Native American Indians used wild onions in a variety of ways, eating them raw or cooked, as a seasoning or vegetable and as medicine. Wild onions were used in syrups, as poultices, as an ingredient in dyes and even as toys. According to diaries of colonists, onion bulbs were planted as soon as they could clear the land in 1648.

The American settlers used wild onions to treat colds, coughs and asthma, and to repel insects. Chinese medicine uses onions to treat angina, coughs, breathing problems and bacterial infections. Onions can improve lung function, especially in asthmatics, and onion extracts are recognized by the World Health Organization (WHO) for providing relief in the treatment of coughs and colds, asthma and bronchitis. Onions are known to decrease bronchial spasms. An onion extract was found to decrease allergy-induced bronchial constriction in asthma patients.

Onions also appear to be useful for the prevention of cardiovascular disease, since they diminish the risk of blood clots. Onions contain a number of sulfides similar to those found in garlic, which may lower blood lipids and blood pressure. Onions are a rich source of flavonoids, substances known to provide protection against cardiovascular disease. The WHO supports the use of onions to prevent atherosclerosis.

Tests have shown that the more pungent varieties of onion appear to possess the greatest amounts of health promoting and infection fighting phytochemicals.

Onion extracts, rich in a variety of sulfides, provide some protection against tumor growth. Studies in Greece have shown a high consumption of onions, garlic and other *Alliums* to be protective against stomach cancer.

Chinese with the highest intake of onions, garlic and other Allium vegetables have a risk of stomach cancer 40 percent less than those with the lowest intake. Elderly Dutch men and women with the highest onion consumption (at least one-half onion/day) had one-half the level of stomach cancer compared with those consuming no onions at all.

Researchers in Russia have confirmed the bactericidal properties of onion. According to Dr. B.P. Tohkin, his studies showed that chewing raw onion for three minutes is sufficient to kill all germs in the mouth.

Onions are noted for providing easily assimilated iron. Onions in the diet can be beneficial in the treatment of anemia.

The onion has long been considered one of the most important aphrodisiac foods and stands second only to garlic. Onion juice mixed with equal amounts of honey is a traditional aphrodisiac remedy in Ayurvedic medicine.

One small cooked onion contains 0.8 grams protein and 1.3 grams of fiber. It also offers potassium, phosphorus, calcium, magnesium, sodium, selenium, vitamin C, folic acid and small amounts of iron, manganese, copper and zinc.

LEEKS - *Allium porrum*

Leeks have long been considered a food of the poor and seen as a symbol of humility. Leeks, rice, almonds and honey was a favorite meal of ancient biblical people. Ancient Egyptians ate their leeks with barley bread, and present day Cherokee people eat the leaves of wild leeks as a spring tonic. Leeks alone, or mixed with honey, is a remedy for sore throat, coughs and colds, and the juice mixed with honey is used to heal wounds.

RAMPS / WILD LEEKS *Allium tricoccum*

Ramps and Wild Leeks are the same plant, a type of wild-growing onion distinguished primarily by growing in different regions.

In the Appalachian range they are known as Ramps, the healer, solace and friend to the mountain people. Ramps are used in folk medicine to keep away cold and flu. They are among the first of the greens to appear in the spring and are used as a traditional spring tonic.

In the North people call the same plant Wild Leeks. High in vitamins C and A, and full of healthful minerals, they have the same cholesterol-lowering properties found in Garlic and other members of the Allium family.

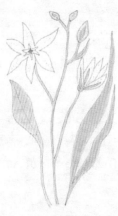

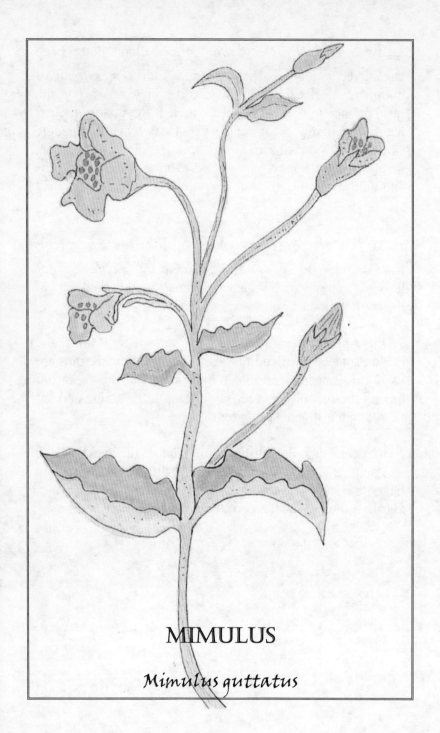

MIMULUS

Mimulus guttatus

THE FIG TREE

Ficus carica,

Ficus sycomorus

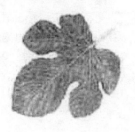

The fig-tree hath put forth her green figs; the vines in flower yield their sweet smell. Canticle 2

Fig trees were likely one of the first cultivated crops and are believed to pre-date the cultivation of wheat, barley and legumes. There is evidence that they were being cultivated more than 11,000 years ago, in the Jordan Valley north of ancient Jericho, at a village known as Gilgal I.

Sycamore figs, *Ficus sycomorus*, were represented on Egyptian tomb walls and reliefs and commonly lined ancient temple gardens. Sometimes referred to as the Egyptian mulberry, the sycamore fig is taller than the common fig and bears a smaller, though sweet and edible, fruit that is produced in racemes. Its heart shaped leaves were used as funerary amulets.

The Egyptian Goddess Hathor was known as "Lady of the Sycamore" and was often depicted pouring a refreshing liquid into the hands of the deceased while their *ba,* or soul, in the form of a bird with a human head, fluttered in nearby branches. Consumption of the fruit was equated with eating the flesh and drinking the blood of Hathor herself.

Egyptian ideas about the sacramental, revitalizing powers of the sycamore fig were known and understood in Canaanite Goddess worship. As we have seen, worshippers of Hathor were among the Hebrews who crossed the Sinai wilderness in search of the Promised Land.

The fig tree is mentioned over fifty times in the Bible and is usually seen as a symbol of nourishment, prosperity and continuity. It was one of the seven fruits of the Promised Land (Deuteronomy 8:8). There is no doubt that figs were a significant part of the diet of ancient civilizations in the Near East and Mediterranean areas.

The juice from both the fruit and leaves of this tree is milky white and was known by the Egyptians as "milk of the sycamore." This medicinal substance was used by them to heal wounds and abscesses. Isaiah found the application of figs beneficial to Hezekiah's boil (2 Kings 20:7; Isaiah 38:21), and the ancient Assyrian's also made use of figs in plasters. The dried fruits contain 50% invert sugar and some sucrose, and these sugars act as healing and "drawing" agents.

`And the trees said to the fig tree, "come you, and reign over us." But the fig tree said to them, "Shall I leave my sweetness and my good fruit?" (Judges 9:10-11).

The common fig we know today, *Ficus carica,* like the olive and the grapevine, has been in cultivation since at least the Early Bronze Age. It is a warm temperate or sub-tropical small tree or shrub, growing to approximately thirty feet, that thrives in hot, arid climates. It originated from the wild figs of the Mediterranean area and is related to many wild species growing in the region toward Afghanistan. There are approximately eight hundred species in the genus *Ficus.*

Fig trees are widespread throughout the Mediterranean lands, beloved by the people here and often seen growing next to homes, in small gardens and even in courtyards. To many, a garden is simply not a garden without a fig tree. The young trees are shrubby with several grey-barked stems and thick twigs, which exude a milky juice when cut.

Leafless in winter, the fig tree bursts its buds in late spring, and its broad, coarse and deeply lobed leaves are fully developed by the summer months.

From the fig tree learn its lesson: as soon as its branch becomes tender and puts forth its leaves, you know that summer is near (Matthew 24:32).

Sumerian tablets record the consumption of common figs in 2,500 B.C. The Greeks believed figs to be a gift of the Goddess Demeter, and Plato documented that athletes at Olympia ate figs to increase their running speed as well as to build strength. Roman Pliny was aware of at least 29 different types of figs. Because of their high sugar content, cooked figs were used as sweeteners in ancient times.

Italians have been eating figs for a very long time. Figs, along with cheese, bread, cabbage and olives, were among the staple foods of the Roman Legions. Many of the immigrants who came to America from Southern Italy, where fig trees grow exceptionally well, planted fig trees where they settled, harvesting the bounty in the summer and covering the trees in the winter when it got cold. I remember my grandfather tending to his fig tree in the lovely garden he and my grandmother shared in back of their brownstone house in Hoboken, New Jersey.

In our village and throughout the Mediterranean, the nourishing, mineral rich fig is regularly consumed both fresh and dried. The delicious fruits offer an abundance of iron, calcium, phosphorus, potassium, protein and fiber. Figs are considered both a food and a medicine that imparts strength and energy to the body and the mind.

Fresh figs can be pale green or a deeper blackish burgundy red, and should look firm and somewhat voluptuous with a bit of roundness to them. If they're overripe they become very sweet and can start to ferment. Some people like this combination of flavors, but others don't. If you buy fresh figs, use them the same day, as they will not last long.

Fresh figs are very perishable. They have a very short shelf life after harvesting and last only about three to five days in refrigeration. Figs that are frozen whole and stored in jars can be expected to last for several months to one year. Figs are easily dried to prolong their storage and then soaked in warm water to restore their shape and softness.

In areas where they grow, figs are generally eaten fresh from the tree and often served with cream and sugar. Fresh figs are usually served at the end of a meal, but sometimes they are combined with thinly sliced prosciutto and presented as an antipasto. Peeled or unpeeled, the fruits are stewed or cooked in various ways, such as in pies, puddings, cakes, bread or other bakery products, and made into ice cream. They are also preserved in sugar syrup or prepared as jam, marmalade, or made into a paste.

In Mediterranean countries, lesser grade figs are fermented into alcohol, and an alcoholic extract of dried figs is used as a flavoring for liqueurs and tobacco.

Much as they were in ancient times, figs are widely used to poultice tumors and other abnormal growths and are considered to be cancer preventive. An extract of figs has been shown to shrink tumors.

Figs also possess antibacterial as well as antiparasitic properties. Both fresh and dried figs are considered astringent, carminative, demulcent as well as nutritive. Syrup of figs is a gentle and effective laxative that is suitable for the young and very old alike.

The lovely leaves of the tree are used to make a perfume with a woodsy aroma called fig-leaf absolute. Fig leaves are added to boiling water and used as a steam bath to ease hemorrhoids, and an infusion of the leaves, as well as the fresh or dried fruit, is consumed to treat diabetes and dissolve calcifications in the kidneys and liver.

The white milky juice of the freshly-broken stalk of a fig tree is applied to the skin to removes warts and is used on ulcers and sores. When dried and powdered, this latex is used to coagulate milk for making cheese. A protein-digesting enzyme, *ficin,* is extracted from it and used for tenderizing meat, rendering fat and clarifying beverages.

The sap was an ingredient in some early commercial household detergents, but its use was discontinued after many reports of irritated or inflamed hands. Fig latex may cause photo-dermatitis. A sunburn-like rash develops when skin that has been in contact with the sap is exposed to ultraviolet light. Photosensitizing compounds related to *furanocoumarin* are thought to be responsible. Workers in commercial orchards wear gloves and protective clothing to guard against the sap.

Fig trees usually bear two crops a year; the early season, or *breba* fruits, which mature in the spring, are considered inferior. Those of the second, or main crop, which matures in late summer, are much more delicious.

Gelato di Fichi - Fig Ice Cream

14 ounces ripe figs, 1/2 cup milk, 1 tablespoon honey and the juice of a lemon. After peeling the figs, blend the pulp with the lemon juice. Combine the milk and honey, and stir them into the figs. Put the mixture into an ice cream maker and enjoy!

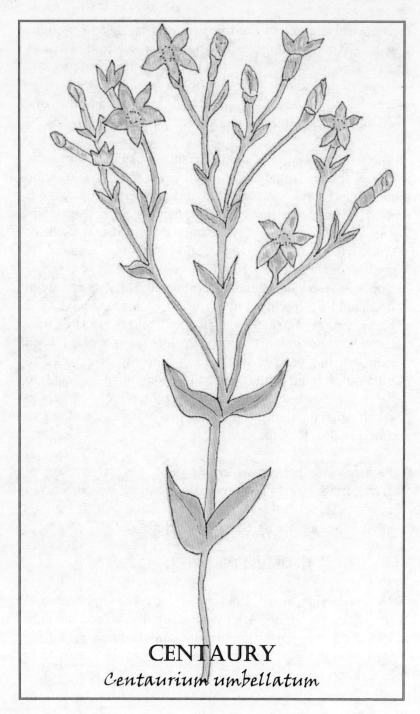

CENTAURY
Centaurium umbellatum

FLOWERS OF FIELD AND GARDEN
OUR LADY'S FLORETTI

A walk around the wild edges of our village, or up into the mountains, delivers a wonderful view of the botanical timelessness of this area. Wild herbs grow abundantly everywhere, as they have for millennia. Every little square of untended earth delivers a magnificent patch of nettles. The hillsides are covered with wild marjoram. The roadsides are matted with chickweed. Borage grows through cracks and crevices, and everywhere huge rosemary bushes grow, laden with dark green needle-like leaves and decorated profusely with delicate sea-blue flowers. Many of the wild herbs that cover the mountain paths are in the mint, or Lamiaceae family.

The LAMIACEAE FAMILY of plants grows naturally and abundantly throughout Southern Italia, as well as the entire Mediterranean region. These wonderful healing plants, such as lavender, sage, rosemary, oregano and marjoram, create a big sensation when in bloom. They are widely cultivated and enjoy a multitude of uses among the people here. In fact, regular use of these common and abundant wild plants has sustained the bodies and minds of a strong and sturdy people through the millennia.

The Lamiaceae family, formerly known as Labiatae, and commonly called the mint family, is a large family of mostly herbs and shrubs that are distributed throughout the world. This family includes many of the well known culinary herbs such as thyme, oregano and basil and lots of abundant wild herbs such as ground ivy and self heal. The plants in the mint family are respected for offering rich stores of minerals, so this is an exceedingly nourishing family of plants.

CHARACTERISTICS:

The plants in this family usually have square stems. The leaves are simple and in pairs up the stem, each pair at right angles to the last, and they are frequently hairy or with scent glands.

The flowers give this plant family its original name of Labiatae. They have two lips, one more protruding than the other (*labia* is the Latin for 'lip'). Generally, the upper lip has two lobes and forms a hood over the lower lip, and the lower lip consists of three lobes which form a landing platform for pollinating insects. The flowers occur in whorls or circles around the stem, and each flower protrudes from a pointed calyx.

Each single flower can produce four seeds. The seeds form at the base of the flower and develop inside the calyx. There is no seed pod. When the seeds are ripe, they simply roll out of the calyx.

The mints get their name from Mintha, the Greek nymph who was transformed into the herb by Persephone when she learned that her husband Pluto had loved the nymph. The Greek word *Heduosmos*, or *mintha,* literally means "having a sweet smell." In Europe the mints were all dedicated to the Virgin Mary. In Italy mint is called *Herba Santa Maria.*

As early as 1550 B.C., the mints were being cultivated in Egyptian gardens and are mentioned in Egyptian and Assyrian medical texts from this time. According to Dioscorides, the Egyptian name for mint was *tis,* and mints were used as a tonic for the stomach. A warm infusion was also given to bring down a fever. Dr. James Duke has posited that this may have been the origin of the word we now use for tea, *tisane.*

Because mint grew so abundantly, the Hebrews banned the sowing and gathering of the mints every seventh year. Mints were widely used as strewing herbs, both in the home and in the temple. Several varieties of mints grew wild in these areas, but horsemint, *Mentha longifolia*, was the most common, and most likely the one mentioned in Matthew and Luke. *"But woe to you Pharisees! For you tithe mint and rue and herbs of all kinds and neglect justice and the love of God."*

The ancient Romans and Greeks also found many uses for the mint family plants. Pliny listed more than forty medicinal uses for the mints. The fragrant leaves were used to impart sweetness and flavor to porridge, added to the Roman baths, invigorated athletes, and bunches of mint were hung in the sick room to speed healing.

DEW OF THE SEA
ROSEMARY

Rosmarinus officinalis

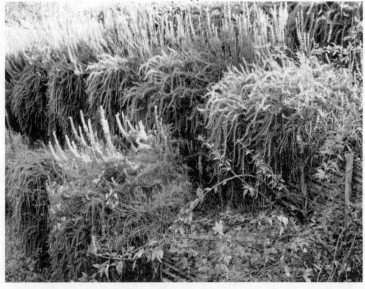

Rosemary is a dearly loved culinary herb throughout the Mediterranean region and deeply respected for its medicinal as well as magical properties. One of the most often used spices in Italian cuisine, rosemary's pungent flavor complements fatty meats particularly well, and many Italian recipes call for rosemary in marinades and as an accent for Mediterranean vegetables, breads, focaccia, soups and pasta.

The Romans planted rosemary in hedges, and the ancient Greeks wove it into crowns to adorn the heads of young women. Ancient legends say that a rosemary bush sheltered the Blessed Mother Mary on her journey into Egypt. Hence it was called afterward Rose of Mary, or rosemary.

Old herbals refer to rosemary as a cure-all, and modern science tells us that it is a supreme cardiac tonic, an energizer for the circulatory system, and will successfully lower blood pressure.

Rosemary is also highly regarded as an antidepressant, nervine, and a restorative tonic for the nervous system. Uplifting and revitalizing, rosemary is a well known brain tonic, clearing the mind and improving memory. Drinking 2 cups of infusion, or taking 30 drops of tincture in water twice daily, is commonly advised when dealing with any of the above, as well as fatigue, exhaustion and stress.

Antioxidant-rich rosemary is often successfully used to help fight infections caused by bacteria and fungi. And rosemary is a welcome stomach tonic. Sipping a warm cup of rosemary tea, or taking 30 drops of tincture in water, eases stomach discomfort and helps relieve gas.

Rosemary also possesses rich stores of analgesic properties. Use the infused oil or liniment to bring blood flow to an area, help ease tense muscles and inflamed joints, and help relieve arthritic/rheumatic conditions. Fresh rosemary tinctured in rubbing alcohol becomes a stimulating liniment known as Queen of Hungary water. This healing liniment was first made in the thirteenth century and was said to have reversed the paralysis of Queen Elizabeth of Hungary, who rubbed it into her legs daily. Rosemary baths, compresses and poultices are similarly therapeutic.

Of course, rosemary is famous for beautiful hair. It's true that the infused oil promotes healthy hair follicles, brings renewed vitality, helps moisturize hair, prevents premature loss and helps to keep the scalp dandruff-free. Apply a bit of rosemary oil to the scalp and hair at least once a week for a head full of beautiful locks.

Rosemary is known as an herb of protection, and I enjoy wrapping it into fragrant smudge sticks to be burned on any occasion.

Rosemary is a perennial plant in warmer climates such as Southern Italy where it grows as a five-or-six-foot-high shrub loaded with blue flowers. Rosemary can be started from seeds or from cuttings.

Gather rosemary any time the leaves are green and vibrant. Strip the dried leaves from the stems for culinary uses, or use the whole sprigs to scent a room, closet or drawer. Tincture rosemary sprigs in 100 proof alcohol, and infuse some in olive oil, rubbing alcohol, vinegar or honey.

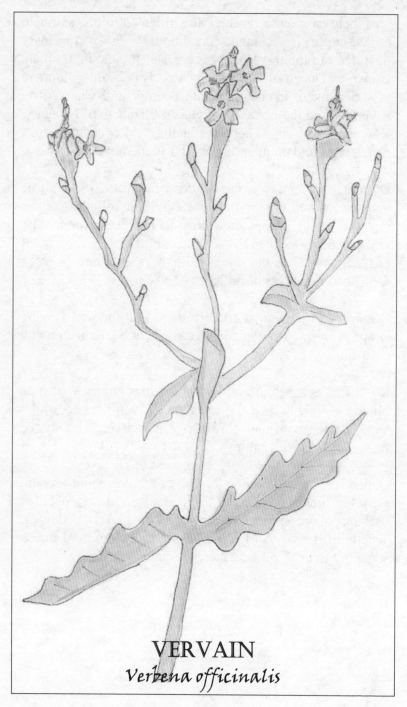

VERVAIN
Verbena officinalis

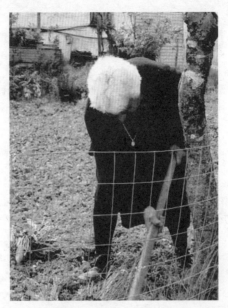

JOY OF THE MOUNTAIN
OREGANO

Origanum vulgare and its cousin wild marjoram, *Origanum majorana*, are both well known and much loved culinary and medicinal spices with ancient roots throughout the Mediterranean.

In the springtime the mountains around Monte San Giacomo become awash in a stunning array of brilliant pinkish purple patches. This is when the wild marjoram blooms. Marjoram has long been referred to as the ***Joy of the Mountain*** - now I know why! The plants are gorgeous, beautiful, sticking out of everywhere, as if the mountains themselves are announcing their happiness that spring has arrived.

Long associated with abundance, fertility and good health, marjoram and oregano made up the herbal wreath that crowned the Mediterranean Mother Goddesses Demeter and Hera. These herbs were also sacred to Venus and Diana and have had a connection to women's health, fertility, strength and vitality down through the ages.

Oregano and wild marjoram promote and encourage the body's production of progesterone. They are excellent hormone balancing allies for both sexes during the menopausal years.

Oregano has powerful antibiotic properties and is strongly active against food-borne pathogens such as *Bacillus cereus, Clostridium, Lactobacillus plantarum* and *Leuconostoc mesenteroides.* Oregano also shows strong activity against a number of other yeasts and fungi and the essential oil kills 100% of the bacteria it contacts. We make a counter wax by adding a bit of beeswax and essential oil to infused oil of oregano. A little bit of this wax rubbed into our cutting board and kitchen work surfaces often, keeps them free of discomfort-causing organisms.

I wish you could taste the delicious pizza my cousins make in their ancient wood-fired oven with a basic dough, fresh tomatoes, homemade mozzarella cheese and plenty of dried oregano!

The dried or fresh leaves of oregano and marjoram are lavishly added to Italian, Spanish, Mexican, Greek and Turkish cuisine.

Add the minced fresh or crushed dried leaves of both marjoram and oregano to sauces, any tomato salad or cooked dish, zucchini or green salads. Oregano spices chili con carne, vegetable soups, onion dishes and barbecue sauces. It is also used to season pork, lamb, fish and chicken.

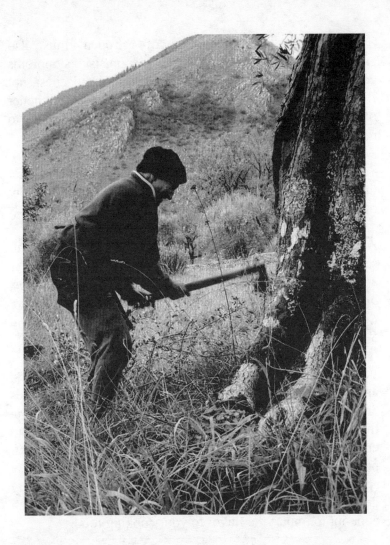

SAGE - *Salvia officinalis* Mediterranean women often use sage, which they call *salvia*, to nourish hormonal production, build strength, enhance vitality and keep their brain functioning well into old age.

Sage is loaded with antioxidants, is anti-aging and offers lots of calcium and magnesium, thujone, flavonoids and phytosterols. It is sedating, soothing, and has a tonic effect on the nerves.

Sage enhances the production of estrogen, thus also enhances fertility and helps ease menopausal symptoms caused by low estrogen levels, such as headaches, hot flashes and night sweats. Sage is a tonic and strengthener of the entire female reproductive system and will help to regulate menstruation and relieve painful cramps.

Sage is also an effective digestive aid; it will help stimulate the appetite and improve digestion by motivating the flow of digestive juices and bile.

A potent broad spectrum antibiotic and immune stimulant, sage possesses antibacterial and antiseptic properties and is active against *Streptococcus pneumoniae, Staphylococcus aureus, Haemophilus influenzae, Pseudomonas aeruginosa, E. coli, Candida albicans, Klebsiella pneumoniae and Salmonella spp.*

Italians fry whole salvia leaves and eat them with potatoes, and often add sage leaves to foccacia. Crush sage leaves and add them to roasts, stews, soups, sauces, chowders, marinades and lima bean dishes. Sprinkle sage leaves to enhance vegetable dishes including onions, eggplant, potatoes and tomato. Sage is also added to cheese, cheese spreads, fish, pork and meat loaf. Sage honey is incredibly delicious. Place fresh sage on top of hot coals during a cookout to impart the flavor to your cooking food.

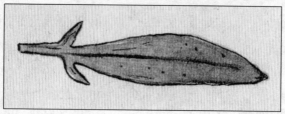

Two more indispensable wild flowers of the fields must be mentioned here. Though not in the Lamiaceae family, both grow abundantly throughout these regions and are widely used by the Mediterranean people.

CHAMOMILE – *Matricaria chamomilla* or *M. matricarioides*

Another delightful and abundant plant that is much loved and well used here in Monte San Giacomo is chamomile. In fact, this herb has long been dedicated to our village patroness Sant Anna (St. Ann), the mother of Mary. The botanical name of the plant, *Matricaria,* derives from the words *mater* and *cara,* meaning dear or beloved mother.

My grandmother used chamomile as a heal-all and offered a cup of its delicate tea to help ease a headache, relieve menstrual cramps, settle upset feelings and as a calming drink after dinner.

Chamomile is very popular and readily available throughout the Mediterranean area. Nerve soothing, anti-inflammatory, antispasmodic, antibacterial, sedative and pain relieving, chamomile has a well deserved reputation as an indispensable healing herb.

In all the little markets as well as the local *farmacia*, or drug store, one finds boxes of chamomile tea for sale. When our friend Reno's cousin Maria, who is studying to be a doctor and is under a great deal of stress, came to visit one day after shopping, she showed me that among her purchases was a box of chamomile tea.

Perhaps best known as an herb to soothe the stomach, chamomile's antispasmodic properties help allay nausea, and it is a well-known emmenagogue.

Traditionally used to help bring on the menses when late, chamomile is also useful for scanty or irregular menstruation and is widely used to ease menopausal discomforts.

An excellent nervine, a nice warm cup of chamomile tea or tincture will help soothe your jangled nerves anytime you are stressed, tense or uptight, and a warm cup before bedtime helps ensure a good night's sleep.

Chamomile makes a wonderfully relaxing bath herb and soothing massage oil. The chamazulene constituent offers a powerful anti-inflammatory effect, and chamomile is one of the most reliable remedies to bring down a fever. The delicate flowers are steeped only 10-20 minutes for a full strength medicinal infusion.

To grow chamomile, simply broadcast the tiny seeds over a well prepared garden bed or pot and press them in. Keep the plot well weeded. Harvest the flowers as they bloom.

POPPIES - *Papaver somniferum, P. rhoeas*

The first time I saw a huge field full of brilliant red corn poppies, I could not believe my eyes. I had never seen such a colorful sight! The delicate red blossoms of the *papavero* waved amid the radiant green wheat grasses for as far as my eyes could see. It was a dazzling welcome to spring.

Poppies have an ancient history of use as medicine. In an Egyptian papyrus written in 1443 B.C., poppy was listed as an important medicine. Its use extended to quieting crying children and healing wounds and boils. The flowers are found in preserved funeral garlands found on Egyptian mummies and were among the items found in eighteenth century dynasty tombs.

Herbalists have long used the petals, leaves and seeds of the poppy as a gentle sedative. A few drops of tincture, or a cup of tea, will have a calming effect, relieve colic, help alleviate insomnia and ease a tension headache.

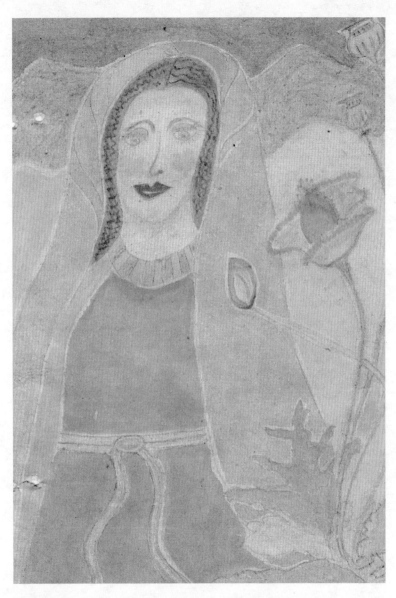

The corn poppy, *Papaver rhoeas*, is used to make a syrup similar to that of rose hips. The red petals are mucilaginous, bitter and expectorant, and their syrup helps alleviate cough and hoarseness. The flower petals possess sedative and pain relieving properties and are occasionally used in soups and in cordials.

California poppy, *Eschscholzia californica,* and *Papaver somniferum* are used in similar ways. *P. somniferum* is thought by some authorities to be the gall added to the vinegar offered to Jesus as he hung on the cross. The plant's species name, *somniferum*, means "sleep inducing."

During the Middle Ages an anesthetic called the "soporific sponge" was widely used. It was usually made with an infusion of poppy, mandrake, hemlock and ivy that was poured over a sponge and held under the patient's nostrils until they fell asleep.

Many plant substances were used to alleviate pain. One of the most commonly used substances was opium derived from the poppy flower, *Papaver somniferum.* Among the other substances used were alcohol or wine, mandrake, belladonna and cannabis.

Opium was very commonly used throughout the 19th century, often as laudanum or tincture of opium, which is a combination of opium and alcohol:

"**Laudanum**: *The common name for Tincture of Opium, and the form in which that drug is most frequently administered. . . is narcotic, sedative, and being made with spirit, is also, to a certain extent, stimulant and antispasmodic. For relieving pain, wherever situated, to diminish irritation, and to procure sleep, it is the best of the medicines we possess.*" *The Family Doctor, a Dictionary of Domestic Medicine and Surgery*, by a Dispensary Surgeon. London, c.1860

Poppy seeds are used in confectionery and in baking a variety of cakes and pastries, such as strudels and Danish pastries. Poppy seed complements honey spread on bread, giving a nice contrast of texture. Fried in butter, poppy seed can be added to noodles or pasta.

Corn poppies have an ancient association with wheat... The red flowers thrive, growing wildly and abundantly, throughout the wheat fields of Europe today, as they have for thousands of years. Their species name *Rhoeas* is Italian and comes from Rhea, the name given to the mother of the founders of Rome, Romulus and Remus. It was also a name attached to Cybele, the Anatolian mother-goddess known as Ceres among the Italic peoples. Ceres, known as Demeter by the Greeks, was the Goddess of Grain.

One ancient legend tells of Rhea (think brilliant red poppies) descending on plains near the Elysian fields in order to console Demeter/Ceres (think vibrant green wheat) after Persephone was lost, and together they bring fertility and growth back to the earth.

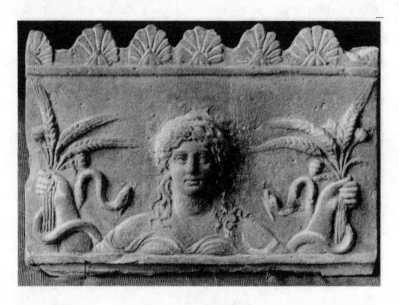

CERES was the ancient Italic goddess of agriculture, grain and bread, the prime sustenance of life. Ceres brought forth the fruits of the resplendent and abundant earth. She was depicted as a mature woman, often crowned with a *corona spicea* (crown of spices) and holding sheaves of wheat and barley. In her image above she emerges from the earth, holding bunches of poppies and grain in her upraised hands while two snakes twine about her arms. Evidence shows that the goddess Ceres was worshiped in Rome as early as 753 B.C.

Virgil claimed that her name was derived from the word *creare*, "to create." Scholars today find the source of her name in the Indo-European *ker*, "to grow," which is the root of *creare*. Her name literally means *growth*.

Ceres was the goddess revered by the early Italic peoples as the very ground from which the crops of grain sprang. She was the bread produced from the grain and the work necessary to raise the crops. Among her many generous gifts to the people were knowledge of the arts of planting and preparing the soil.

The first fruits of the harvest were offered to Ceres, and those who grew or worked with grain honored her with votive inscriptions and offerings.

Ceres presided over the *frumentationes*, the distribution of grain to the urban poor, and the *annona*, the administration of the Roman grain supply. She was associated with the rural areas and the people who lived there. Some of her traditional epithets include:

flava, golden color of grain; *frugifera*, bearer of crops; *larga*, abundant; *fecunda*, fecund; *fertilis*, fertile; *genetrix frugum*; progenetress of the crops and *potens frugum*, powerful in crops

Only later, after she became part of the Aventine Triad with Liber and Libera, does Ceres begin to assimilate the mythology and iconography of the Greek Demeter, including the symbols of the Eleusinian Mysteries, into her cult. Romans participated in the Eleusinian mysteries in the name of their revered goddess Ceres. On coins issued in the second century B.C., Ceres is depicted with symbols of the Mysteries, such as riding in a chariot drawn by snakes while holding a torch in her right hand.

Ceres was associated not only with the fertility and fecundity of the earth and abundant crops of grain but with women's fertility and childbearing as well. As *Ceres Mater*, she was the Goddess of Motherhood, a concept cherished by the Italians. Reliefs from the imperial period show Ceres attending at the birth of Apollo and Diana.

Ceres' major festival was the Cerealia, held on April 19 to celebrate the growth of grain and other agricultural products. The oldest ritual of this festival, held at the Circus Maximus, was tying lit torches to the tails of foxes who would then run wildly through the fields. This ancient magical rite was enacted yearly to stir up the energy of young green growth and to stimulate protection for the crops.

In 176 B.C. *ludi scaenici*, or dramatic productions, were added to the festival. These were enacted as an offering to the Goddess, beseeching her to look kindly on the people and give them a good harvest.

The goddess Flora, who governed the blooming of plants, was closely associated with Ceres. Ceres is also sometimes identified with Gaia. Later, as Christianity spread through the lands, Ceres became Mary...

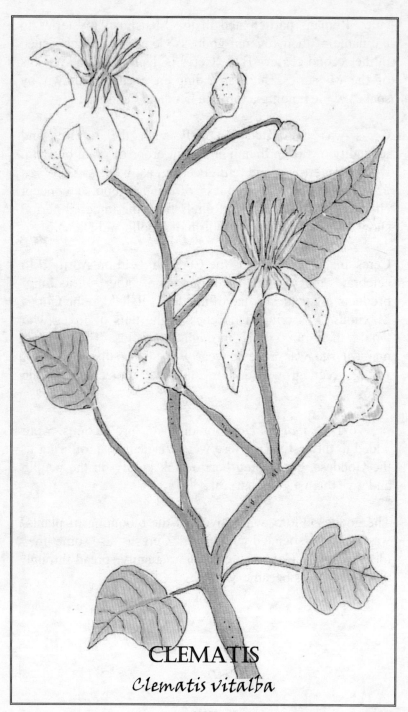

CLEMATIS
Clematis vitalba

ASSUMPTION DAY
FIRST-FRUITS FESTIVAL

The special flower of this day is the fragrant virgin's bower, Clematis virginiana.

The Feast of the Assumption of the Blessed Virgin Mary is celebrated by Catholics on August 15th. This day, in honor of Mary being received into heaven and crowned as Queen, evolved from ancient traditional harvest celebrations held at this time of year, the annual blessing of fruits, herbs and flowers.

Mary is our first fruit,
the first fruit of the new covenant.

She assumed the role previously played by Hecate and Artemis, both of whom were honored on the full moon of August as the protectress of herbs, flowers and fruits, and particularly of grapes and grain. In ancient days the calendar was based on lunar phases and each month began with the new moon, thus August 15 would have fallen on a full moon.

The Feast of the Assumption was proclaimed a special feast day in honor of the Blessed Mother in 600 A.D. in the East, and was adopted approximately 50 years later in the West.

The story of Mary's Assumption comes from ancient stories called the Obsequies of the Holy Virgin, which were written in Syria at the beginning of the third century. One of these stories, called "The Departure of My Lady Mary from this World," describes how Mary's body was lifted up into Heaven.

These early stories say that Mary's Assumption took place at Ephesus, where she lived under the care of the apostle

John. Ephesus was the site of one of the most renowned sanctuaries of Artemis and the home of her well-known statue with many breasts, symbolizing the productive and nurturing powers of the earth. Our Mary, well known for nurturing and protecting, clearly carried on this role.

And the apostles also ordered that there should be a commemoration of the Blessed One on the thirteenth Ab (August), on account of the vines bearing bunches of grapes and on account of the trees bearing fruit, that clouds of hail, bearing stones of wrath, might not come, and the trees be broken and the vines with their clusters...

In the East, where the Assumption Feast has its roots, the day is still commemorated with elaborate ceremonies for the blessing of fruit trees and grain. In modern Syria, both Moslems and Christians celebrate the Feast of the Assumption in similar ways. They make bouquets of newly harvested wheat and bake small triangular cakes. These gifts are graciously offered to the Virgin Mother, as was the way of their ancestors for many millennia before Mary.

In many Catholic countries throughout Europe, Assumption Day still marks the period for invoking blessings on vineyards, herbs and grain. Traditionally, freshly gathered herbs are carried to the church on this day to be blessed and then used for medicine and healing or bound into a sheaf and hung in the home all year to protect against infirmity.

Throughout central Europe, this feast was also known as Our Lady's Herb Day and it marked the start of *Our Lady's 30 Days*, a period of special benevolence lasting for one full month. During this time animals and plants were believed to lose any harmful qualities and all foods were considered wholesome. This period of munificence coincides with the *Weeks of Comfort*, seven weeks following the full moon in the Jewish month of Av during which the spiritual readings are comforting, promising peace and prosperity.

Armenian communities all over the world still bless grapes on Assumption Day and also celebrate it as the name day feast of all the local women and girls named Mary. Large trays piled high with freshly harvested grapes are carried to church to receive the blessings of the priest. After Mass the people assemble in the vineyards to eat grapes and celebrate the village Marys.

When Pope Pius XII proclaimed the Assumption an article of faith in 1950, Carl Jung perceived it as a critical juncture in Western culture; the image of the divine feminine was coming back into the light. The Queen of Heaven was being acknowledged once again in the West.

In Greece, the Assumption is called the *Dormition* or *Kimesis* (Sleeping), and is the most important of the summer holidays. During this full month devoted to Mary her icons depict her dead on a bier, with Christ behind her, holding her soul in his arms like an infant.

One description of the Kimesis celebration as held at Kefallonia tells of snakes called "the snakes of the Virgin," slithering over the sacred icons, the offerings and the people in the congregation.

"Each day I visit black Mary, who looks at me with her wise face, older than old and ugly in a beautiful way...she is a muscle of love, this Mary. I feel her in unexpected moments, her Assumption into heaven happening in places inside of me. She will suddenly rise, and when she does, she does not go up, up into the sky, but further and further inside of me. August says she goes into the holes life has gouged out of us." Sue Monk Kidd

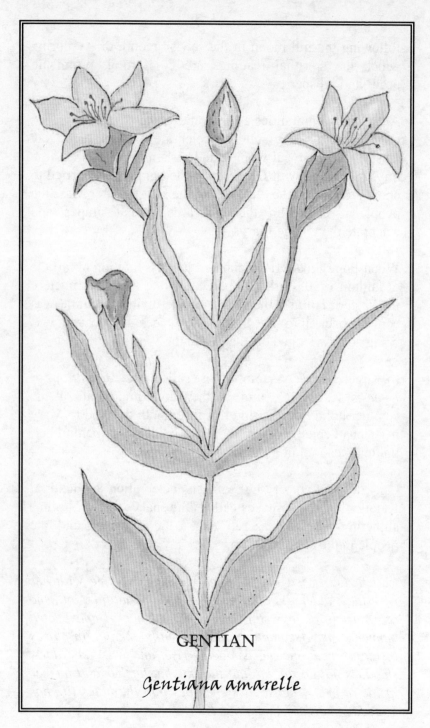

GENTIAN

Gentiana amarelle

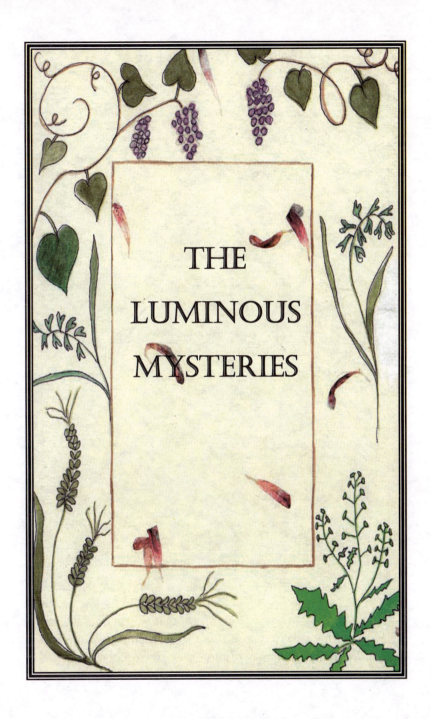

THE LUMINOUS MYSTERIES

LUMINOUS MYSTERIES

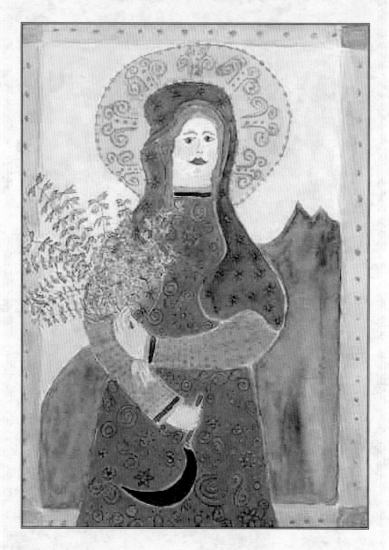

The Luminous Mysteries highlight grains, such as wheat, oats, barley and rye, grapes and fermented food and drink and the Brassica family plants, such as broccoli, mustard and radish.

THE STAFF OF LIFE

Recently scientists working in the flooded ruins of an ancient fishing camp in Israel found evidence that the residents were collecting wild grain, pounding it into flour and possibly baking bread at least 10,000 years before the advent of cultivated crops.

Traces of barley and other grains were detected in the seams of a grinding stone unearthed at Ohalo II, a settlement on the southwest shore of the Sea of Galilee that thrived 22,000 years ago. This discovery is the oldest evidence found of humans processing cereal grains.

Besides the milled grain there was also considerable evidence of charred or parched grains at the site, especially smaller seeds, suggesting that the ancient residents may have gathered cereal to make gruel.

Agriculture, practiced by settled peoples cultivating crops, began to appear between 10,000 and 12,000 years ago in disparate cultures in the Middle East, the Far East and Mesoamerica.

In the book *Noah's Flood,* Columbia University marine geologists William Ryan and Walter Pitman III build the case of a catastrophic flood in the Black Sea causing local Stone Age settlers to move along with their farming skills to dry lands in Europe and Asia. Using archeological, geological, and climate data to support their claim, they posit that the flood that inspired the Epic of Gilgamesh and the story of Noah may also have spurred a global farming revolution.

Ancient civilizations such as Egyptian, Babylonian, Greek, Cretan and Roman were highly dependent on wheat and barley as their principal foods. Einkorn, Emmer,

Khorasan/Kamut and Spelt are among the earliest cultivated wheats and are usually referred to as "ancient wheats."

These ancient wheats represent a rich source of genetic diversity and their cultivation has survived on a limited scale in Italy, Switzerland, Germany and Poland to this day. During the past two decades the conservation and green movements in Europe have promoted cultivation of ancient wheats in an effort to preserve genetic resources. And in the United States there is now a groundswell of interest in growing these ancient wheats in home gardens. In Maine, FEDCO member Eli Rugosa is working in this field.

At present most of the wheats grown around the world are hybrids that have been created from ancient wheats over the past 100 to 150 years.

The process of domestication and breeding of the ancient grains may have produced varieties of wheat with particular characters, such as higher yielding and better disease resistance. However, the hybrids may lack some of the other unique properties of the ancestral wheats, such as nutrient content.

For instance, einkorn was found to contain significantly higher level of lutein compared with other wheat species. Lutein reduces the risk of age-related macular degeneration (AMD) and cataracts and protects against heart disease and cancer.

Ancient wheats have been used for the treatment of a wide range of health conditions, such as ulcerative colitis, elevated cholesterol, hypertension, diabetes, rheumatoid arthritis, depression and cancer.

POACEAE FAMILY OR GRAMINEAE

The fossil record tells us that the plants in this family, called grasses, evolved around 65 million years ago. There are approximately 600 genera and between 9,000-10,000 species in the Poaceae family, which is one of the oldest of the plant families.

Plant communities dominated by Poaceae are called grasslands and, depending on their location, pampas, plains, steppes, or prairie. It is estimated that grasslands comprise between 20 - 30% of the vegetation cover of the earth.

The Poaceae family is the most important of all plant families to human economies: it includes the staple food grains grown around the world, lawn and forage grasses, and bamboo, widely used for construction throughout Asia.

CHARACTERISTICS:

Grasses have hollow stems that are plugged at intervals called **nodes**. Their leaves are alternate, distichous (in one plane) and sometimes spiral, parallel-veined and arise at the nodes. The leaf blades of many grasses are hardened with silica which helps discourage grazing animals. In some grasses the silica creates leaf blades sharp enough to cut human skin. Grass blades grow at the base of the blade and not from the tips.

The flowers of Poaceae are typically arranged in a terminal panicle or spike and made of many small spikelets, each having one or more florets. The fruit is called a caryopsis.

The success of the grasses lies in their unique growth processes and in their amazing diversity.

Agricultural grasses grown for their edible seeds are called cereals. Three cereals in particular, wheat, corn and rice, provide more than half of all calories eaten by humans and 70% of all crops grown are grasses. Cereals constitute the major source of carbohydrates for humans and perhaps the major source of protein.

Sugar cane, another plant in this family, is the major source of sugar production. Many other grasses are grown for forage and animal food. Grasses are used as food plants by many species of butterflies and moths.

Grasses are strong and useful. Scaffolding made from bamboo is able to withstand typhoon force winds that would break steel scaffolding. Large bamboos are strong and stout and can be used in a manner similar to timber. Bamboo is also used to make innumerable tools and implements. Grass fibers are used to make paper and for bio-fuel.

Cereals and legumes were domesticated in tandem: wheat, barley, pea, lentil, broad bean and chick pea cultivation was widespread throughout southern Europe and parts of Asia in 4,000 B.C.

wheat, barley, rye, oats, sorghum, corn, rice, millet, spelt, lemongrass

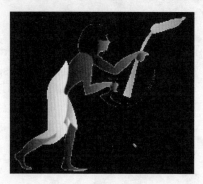

In 8,000 B.C., people in the Fertile Crescent of the Near and Middle East (Syria, Iran, Iraq, Turkey, Jordan and Israel today) were cultivating wheats, barley, lentils, peas, bitter vetch and chick-peas.

The archaeological evidence reveals that the wheats, and some of the legumes, had reached Greece by 6,000 B.C. The Neolithic cultures of Thessaly and Crete were cultivating wheat, barley and lentils by this time also. Evidence of the presence of wheat has been found in the Danube Basin, the Nile valley, and the Indian subcontinent around this same time.

Harvested grain was crushed by hand using a simple mortar and pestle. The Egyptians developed the first grinding stone, called a *quern*. The earliest breads were unleavened and made from a mixed variety of grains. They resembled Indian chapattis and Mexican tortillas.

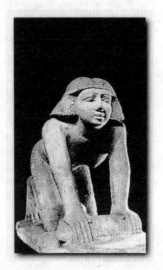

The Egyptians developed grain production along the fertile Nile River between 5,000-3,500 B.C. By 3,000 B.C., tougher wheat varieties were being developed and bread baking was a respected skill along with brewing beer. In the warm Egyptian climate, wild yeasts were attracted to the multi-grain flour mixtures and bakers were experimenting with leavened dough.

The Egyptians invented the closed oven, and bread assumed great significance among them. Homage was paid to Osiris, their god of grain. Bread was used as currency, and the workers who built the pyramids were paid in loaves of bread.

Grain was a significant staple food, and its cultivation spread to the Balkans, throughout Europe, and eventually reached Britain and Scandinavia by 4,000-2,000 B.C. The first iron ploughshares were being pulled by horses by 1,500 B.C. Approximately five hundred years later the south of England had become an agricultural center. Barley and oats were widely grown, and wheat became a key crop soon after.

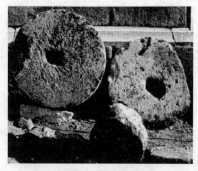

Natural leavened breads were popular among the Romans in 1,000 B.C., and by 500 B.C. they had developed their own milling quern: a round stone wheel turned on a second wheel that was fixed. This Roman design was the basis of all milling until the industrial revolution in the 19th century and is still the way stone ground flour is produced today.

The first bakers' guilds were formed in Rome by 150 B.C., and it was a Roman who invented the first mechanical dough-mixer, which was powered by horses and donkeys in 55 B.C.

Clearly grains have provided humans (and many animals) with an essential part of their diet since prehistoric times when Paleolithic peoples gathered seeds and crushed them for gruels and porridge. All grains are excellent sources of complex carbohydrates, offer a wealth of vitamins and minerals, antioxidants and phytosterols and are naturally low in fat.

Each whole kernel of grain is a storehouse of nutrients essential to the human diet.

Whole grains haven't had their bran and germ removed by milling, making them better sources of fiber. Among many health benefits, a high-fiber diet also tends to make a meal feel more filling so you stay full for a longer time.

When milling grains to produce flour, many of the most nutritious parts are eliminated in exchange for a white color and better keeping qualities.

Refined wheat flour, or white flour, is usually enriched with vitamins and minerals to approach the original content of the grain. But many nutrients, especially those found in parts of the kernel that are eliminated during the refining process, are not replaced. Antioxidants and other phytonutrients necessary for the prevention of many diseases are lost.

Barley, Brown Rice, Buckwheat (Kasha), Bulgur (cracked Wheat), Millet, Oatmeal, Popcorn, Whole-wheat Bread, Pasta or Crackers, Wild Rice

Whole grain flour includes all three parts of the grain kernel: the exterior part of the grain called the bran, the germ and the endosperm. White flour contains just the endosperm, which is the largest part of the grain.

The *endosperm* is about 83 percent of the kernel weight. The endosperm contains the greatest share of the protein in the whole kernel, carbohydrates, iron as well as many B-complex vitamins, such as riboflavin, niacin and thiamine.

Bran is approximately 14 ½ percent of the kernel weight. Bran is included in whole wheat flour and is available separately. Of the nutrients in whole wheat, the bran contains a small amount of protein, larger quantities of the B-complex vitamins, trace minerals, and indigestible cellulose material.

The *germ* makes up 2 ½ percent of the kernel weight. The germ is the embryo or sprouting section of the seed and is usually separated because of the fat, which because of the possibility of rancidity, limits the storage time of the flour. Of the nutrients in whole wheat, the germ contains minimal quantities of protein, but a greater share of B-complex vitamins and trace minerals.

Eating a variety of whole grains not only ensures that you get more nutrients, but also helps make your meals and snacks more interesting. And remember to soak or sprout your grains prior to cooking.

Grains contain phytic acid, a naturally occurring substance in the outer layer of the bran that blocks the absorption of important nutrients such as iron, zinc, copper, calcium and vitamin B12. Soaking or sprouting your grains will help to break down and neutralize this acid, making the grains much more nourishing and digestible. During the soaking and fermenting process the gluten and other hard to digest proteins in grains are also partially broken down into simpler and more readily absorbable compounds.

In fact, according to Sally Fallon, author of *Nourishing Traditions,* grains containing gluten, such as oats, rye and especially wheat, should not be consumed unless they have first been either soaked (for at least several hours or overnight), or fermented. Rice, millet and buckwheat do not contain gluten and are more easily digested, so soaking is not necessary.

A diet rich in properly prepared whole grains not only satisfies hunger and taste but can protect against the development of many chronic diseases, including cancer, cardiovascular disease and diabetes. In addition, whole grains in the diet provide good, stable energy and endurance, calm and steady the nerves and support sound sleep. Whole grains will also help keep elimination moving regularly, improve reflexes and enhance memory and thinking processes.

Chinese medicine says that grains support the process of finding the *Golden Mean,* or the place of receptivity, relaxation and mental focus.

OTHER VITAMINS AND MINERALS IN GRAINS

Thiamine - B vitamin needed daily for good appetite, digestion and strong, steady nerves.

Niacin - A B vitamin essential for the efficient use of protein by the body. Also, critically important for healthy brain function.

Riboflavin - Essential for the respiration and health of every cell; combines with protein to ensure oxygen-rich blood; necessary for good eyesight.

Zinc - Important for skin healing, growth, reproductive health and fertility.

Trace Minerals - Whole grains are a good source of selenium and magnesium, nutrients essential to good health.

Iron - Builds vitality, nourishes the blood.

WHEAT *Triticum aestivum* is cooling by nature,
with a sweet and salty flavor. Wheat absorbs a wider range of nutrients from the soil than other grains, and its nutrient

profile is similar to that of the human body. It has been considered the ideal food for human growth and development.

In Chinese medicine wheat is thought to nourish the heart-mind. *"It calms and focuses the mind and can be used for palpitations, insomnia, irritability, menopausal distress and emotional instability. It encourages growth, weight gain and fat formation – and is especially good for children and frail people."* Paul Pitchford, Healing with Whole Foods

Wheat sometimes incites an allergic reaction, especially when the flour is rancid. Wheat needs to be used soon after grinding, or kept cool, in an airtight container, and used within two weeks. Some people are allergic only to processed wheat products and do fine with pre-soaked or sprouted wheat. If you suffer from wheat allergies, avoid it.

Paul Pitchford explains that many people are allergic to this vital food because of over eating refined and rancid wheat products that have been bred for smut resistance continuously since 1926. The "new and improved" wheat species of today are simply not the same as the so-called *ancient wheats* of our ancestors. Try to obtain organically grown wheat and wheat products if possible.

WHEATGRASS Charles F. Schnabel, an agricultural chemist, first experimented with young grasses in 1930, when he used fresh cut grass in an attempt to nurse dying hens back to health. The hens not only recovered, but they produced eggs at a higher rate than healthy hens.

Encouraged by these results, he began drying and powdering grass for his family and neighbors to supplement their diets.

After further experiments with the grasses, during which his chickens doubled their egg production, Schnabel started promoting his discovery to feed mills, chemists and the food industry. By 1940, cans of Schnabel's powdered grass were on sale in major drug stores throughout the United States and Canada.

Ann Wigmore contributed to the popularization of wheatgrass in the 1940s. When Wigmore was a child, she observed her grandmother helping WWI soldiers heal their wounds using local herbs. As an adult, she developed colon cancer and faced the loss of both legs after a traffic accident shattered them. Her doctors wanted to amputate her legs when gangrene set in. Wigmore refused and was determined to heal herself using natural means. She discarded her typical American diet for one that focused on vegetables, grains, seeds and greens. She poulticed her gangrene feet with wild herbs. Realizing winter was approaching and fresh greens would not be available, she prayed for inspiration.

"I asked God for direction. He supplied an exciting solution. The use of grains to grow greens in the kitchen." Dr. Ann Wigmore

She recovered from both her cancer and her wounds. She attributed her success to the wheat grass and shared her discovery by writing several books and creating a school. Believing that most people would not chew grass, Wigmore modified a small meat grinder and developed the first wheatgrass juicer. This made it possible for anyone to grow wheatgrass and juice it in their homes.

Schnabel's research was conducted with wheatgrass grown outdoors in Kansas. His wheatgrass required 200 days of slow growth, through the winter and early spring. It was harvested at the jointing, or reproductive stage, when the plant reached its peak nutritional potential. Schnabel's research showed that after jointing, concentrations of chlorophyll, protein and vitamin decline sharply. His harvested grass was dehydrated and made into powders and tablets for human and animal consumption. Wheatgrass grown indoors in trays for ten days contains similar nutritional content.

The recommended dosage is 30 ml once daily. For therapeutic benefits, 2–4 oz. is taken 1-3 times daily on an empty stomach before meals. Some people experience nausea on high dosages of wheatgrass

Nutrient comparison of 1 oz. of wheatgrass juice, broccoli and spinach.

Nutrient	Wheatgrass Juice	Broccoli	Spinach
Protein	860 mg	800 mg	810 mg
Beta carotene	120 IU	177 IU	2658 IU
Vitamin E	880 mcg	220 mcg	580 mcg
Vitamin C	1 mg	25.3 mg	8 mg
Vitamin B_{12}	0.30 mcg	0 mcg	0 mcg
Phosphorus	21 mg	19 mg	14 mg
Magnesium	8 mg	6 mg	22 mg
Calcium	7.2 mg	13 mg	28 mg
Iron	0.66 mg	0.21 mg	0.77 mg
Potassium	42 mg	90 mg	158 mg

Wheatgrass is believed to have a beneficial effect on the digestive system, help prevent cancer, diabetes and stroke, alleviate constipation, assist in detoxifying heavy metals in the blood stream, nourish the liver and promote well being.

To "break bread" with one's neighbor is to become intimate. Breaking bread is an ancient ritual ~ it means sharing what we have. Stu Silverstein, Bread on Earth

Although grinding grain results in some loss of nutrients, the natural leavening process reintroduces many vitamins and enzymes by fermentation, and more than that, creates a well integrated, living, breathing substance of nourishment. Substantial sustenance.

Bread, and especially leavened breads such as sourdough breads, are exceedingly wholesome and nutritious. Eaten with well made soup, cooked or raw vegetable combinations, or with a spread such as organic butter or cheese, bread provides a good portion of the nutrients of any simple, healthy, well balanced meal.

Sourdough and natural leavening have been used for many thousands of years. Yeast is a relatively new invention and was discovered in a chemistry lab about 100 years ago.

Naturally leavened bread is thought by many to be nutritionally superior to yeasted breads, which can cause bloating, intestinal disturbances, a proliferation of yeast overgrowth, and exacerbation of neurological and degenerative conditions.

The longer proofing of naturally leavened breads provides time for the fermenting process to release more nutrients into the dough and the natural bacterial action as well as the baking process neutralize almost all of the phytic acid in the grain. Furthermore, naturally leavened breads actually improve with age! They get better and even more nourishing five to ten days after being made and can be stored for several weeks.

WHEAT FLOURS

WHOLE WHEAT FLOUR is a coarse-textured flour ground from the entire wheat kernel and thus contains the bran, germ and endosperm. The presence of bran reduces gluten development. Baked products made from whole wheat flour tend to be heavier and denser than those made from white flour.

Whole wheat flour is a good source of *complex carbohydrates,* the most efficient source of energy available to the human body and also the single most deficient item in the typical modern diet. It also offers *fiber,* the indigestible carbohydrate in food that acts like a broom to sweep out the digestive tract. Wheat foods are moderate sources of *incomplete protein.* This means that while wheat and other cereal grains may contain all eight of the amino acids necessary for good health, not all eight are found at adequate levels.

However, combining wheat or other cereal grains with animal proteins or legumes makes the grain protein complete. Within the cereal group, wheat contains more protein than rice or corn. It is interesting to note that the cultivation of grains and beans (legumes) took place in tandem in all areas of the world where they are both grown.

ALL-PURPOSE FLOUR is the finely ground endosperm of the wheat kernel separated from the bran and germ during the milling process. All-purpose flour is made from hard wheats or a combination of soft and hard wheat. It's used to bake yeast breads, cakes, cookies, pastries and noodles.

ENRICHED ALL-PURPOSE FLOUR has iron and B-vitamins added in amounts equal to or exceeding that of whole wheat flour.

BLEACHED ENRICHED ALL-PURPOSE FLOUR is treated with chlorine to mature the flour, condition the gluten and improve the baking quality.

UNBLEACHED ENRICHED ALL-PURPOSE FLOUR is bleached by oxygen in the air during an aging process and is off-white in color. Nutritionally, bleached and unbleached flour are the same.

BREAD FLOUR, from the endosperm of the wheat kernel, is milled primarily for commercial bakers but is also available at retail stores. It is similar to all-purpose flour, but has greater gluten strength and generally is used for yeast breads.

CAKE FLOUR is milled from soft wheat, and is especially suitable for cakes, cookies, crackers and pastries.

PASTRY FLOUR is milled from a soft, low gluten wheat and is comparable in protein but lower in starch than cake flour.

GLUTEN FLOUR is used by bakers with flours having a low protein content because it improves the baking quality and produces gluten bread of high protein content.

SEMOLINA is the coarsely ground endosperm of durum wheat, is high in protein and is used in quality pasta products.

DURUM FLOUR is a by-product of semolina production and is used to make commercial U.S. noodles.

FARINA is the coarsely ground endosperm of hard wheat and is the prime ingredient in many U.S. breakfast cereals and pasta.

BARLEY *Hordeum vulgare* is cooling, sweet and salty in flavor and very easily digested. It is often made into a thin soup for convalescents. Whole barley, or what is called sproutable barley, is much more nutritious than pearl barley, which is more commonly available. Whole barley has twice the calcium, triple the iron and 25% more protein according to Paul Pitchford, who uses barley soup or cream cereal made from barley flour to *"treat diarrhea, soothe inflamed membranes, alleviate painful urination, quell fever and reduce swellings and tumors."*

Flat barley cakes or breads were a favorite of the ancient Egyptians. Barley flour makes a sticky bread and is usually mixed half and half with wheat flour for lightness.

BUCKWHEAT *Fagopyrum esculentum* Sweet and neutral buckwheat improves the appetite and strengthens the intestines. Rutin, a bioflavonoid found in abundance in buckwheat, strengthens capillaries and blood vessels, helps reduce blood pressure and increases circulation to the hands and feet. Rutin is an effective protector against the effects of x rays and other forms of radiation. And young buckwheat greens are an excellent source of chlorophyll, vitamins and enzymes.

Buckwheat makes a dark, heavy, substantial bread. It's often combined with wheat and rice flours.

CORN *(Maize) Zea mays* This native grain of the Americas is sweet and diuretic. It nourishes the heart, improves the appetite, helps regulate digestion, promotes healthy gums and teeth and helps alleviate sexual dysfunction. In native cultures corn was traditionally cooked with a bit of lime which provides the niacin that corn is nearly completely missing. It seems all ancient indigenous people knew about food combinations...

Great Corn Mother, or Panchamama, Goddess of the Crops, is an ancient South American Mother. The Aztecs call her Chicomecoatlis. Her name means seven serpents and the digging stick used for planting seeds. Among the Pueblo people seven ears of corn were presented to Corn Mother each summer by three girls representing three phases of a growing plant; sprout, growth and maturity. This mother wore a blue skirt covered with white flowers, her face was painted with red ochre, her shield emblazoned with the sun. She carried a knife of obsidian in her hand. She was the first mother of Mexico.

The blue corn that the Hopi and Navajo people grow has been a staple food for them for many centuries. It provides more than 20% more protein, 50% more iron and double the magnesium and potassium of white or yellow corn. Corn meal makes a nice yellow bread with a wonderful texture.

Corn silk is a soothing diuretic, and a daily cup or two of tea or 20-30 drops of tincture in water is used to alleviate urinary problems and kidney stones.

MILLET *Pennisetum glaucum* Cooling, sweet and salty, especially rich in amino acids and silicon, millet's alkalinizing nature eases overly acid conditions and helps to sweeten the breath. It possesses antifungal properties and regular consumption discourages overgrowth of *Candida albicans*. Millet has been called the queen of the grains and is recommended to prevent morning sickness and ease digestive upsets, indigestion and vomiting.

Millet flour is combined with other flours for best results. Combine 1/3 millet with 2/3 whole wheat.

OATS *Avena sativa*

Sweet and warming, restorative oats in the diet assure strong nerves, calm steady mind, good coordination and balance, excellent reproductive functioning, healthy sex drive, strong heart and circulatory system, strong bones, balanced hormones, low cholesterol and normal blood pressure. Oats have the most magnesium of any plant, offer abundant silicon and calcium, a slew of B complex vitamins, lots of phytosterols, and vitamin E.

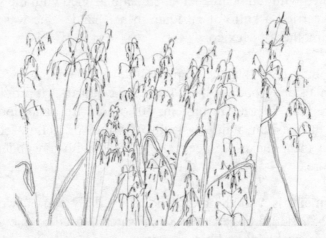

Plenty of magnesium in the diet is implicated in a lessening of the swelling and pain of osteoarthritis and other painful joint disorders. In addition, magnesium assures the best absorption of the abundant calcium in oats and helps relax the muscles. Magnesium is necessary for the electrical body to function optimally, for the heart to beat regularly, and for that elusive quality known as magnetism.

Oat plants harvested in the flowering milky stage and then dried are known as oatstraw. Oatstraw refers to both the flowering tops and the stem of the plant and is used to make wonderfully nourishing and delicious herbal infusions. Oatstraw infusions are a great way to get the benefits of oats. Drinking 2-4 cups daily imparts all the benefits of eating oats and is especially hormonal balancing, grounding and vitality building.

There is an old saying having to do with "feeling your oats," meaning feeling frisky and full of good energy. That's oats.

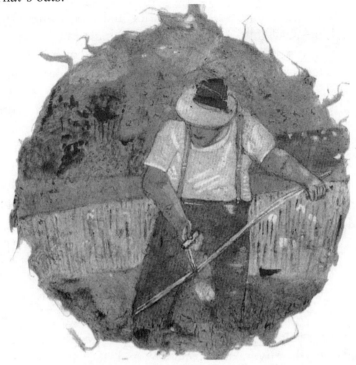

Oat flour is light and airy and adds moisture to cakes and pastry. It can be substituted for pastry flour, and about 20% can be added to whole wheat, rice and corn flours.

RICE *Oryza sativa* is a tropical grain, sweet and soothing to the stomach. Rice provides an abundance of B complex vitamins, is strengthening to the nervous system and helps alleviate depression. It is a hypoallergenic grain. Whole grain rice is brown rice and is far superior to white rice, which is missing the bran and its fiber, the germ and its oils and the other nutrients found in these parts. An ancient Japanese proverb says that eating grains without their skins causes people to become poor and to have no clothes.

Mochi is made with sweet rice and is easy to digest and especially nourishing for nursing mothers, those recovering from illness, and anyone in a weakened condition. It's made by pounding well cooked rice and then forming the resulting paste into balls or patties, which can be served fresh or stored for later use. The patties will harden after 12 hours and can then be pan fried, baked or boiled into soup.

Wild rice is not a true rice but more closely related to corn. It was known as "water grass" or *manomen* to the native tribes of the Minnesota area among who it was a staple food. Wild rice is a hardy food for a cold climate, has more protein than any other rice and offers lots of B vitamins and an abundance of minerals. It is said to concentrate warmth in the interior of the body.

Rice flour blends well with other flours, and adding 20% of it to other flours makes a sweeter and smoother bread.

RYE *Secale cereale* is hard and bitter and a perfect grain for sourdough breads. Because of its bitter quality, it benefits the liver, the pancreas and the spleen. Raw, sprouted or soaked, it provides fluorine, necessary for strong teeth enamel, hair and nails. It is an excellent grain for cold, harsh climates.

According to Paul Pitchford, rye is a potent healing grain and its use has been neglected. *"This cereal grain in its whole form, cool-milled on stone and with all of its bran kept intact, has the capability of reducing and totally eliminating vessel and plaque calcification. Rye also possesses the power to re-energize anemic bodies and rebuild the entire digestive system."*

Rye was the major ingredient in the breads made by the poor during the Medieval times. It was often mixed with flours made from wildgathered substances, such as acorns and horse chestnuts.

Ergot is a fungus, *Claviceps purpurea* that grows on some grains, but especially on rye. Because of this, rye is largely ignored. Ergot contains poisonous alkaloids, one of which is lysergic acid, thought to have been the cause of St. Anthony's fire, which plagued people who ate contaminated rye during the Middle Ages. It is important to know the source of your rye, and to obtain an assurance that it is free of ergot. However, the natural leavening process completely neutralizes ergots' alkaloid substances.

Rye flour makes a dense, sticky bread and can be combined in equal parts with either rice or whole wheat flour for a lighter loaf.

SPELT *Triticum spelta* is a sweet, moistening, warming cousin of wheat. Originally from Southeast Asia, it arrived in the Middle East 9,000 years ago and spread across Europe.

Hildegard of Bingen said that spelt was the best grain for the human body. It contains gluten, but is often well tolerated by those with gluten sensitivity, including those with celiac disease. Spelt is densely packed with nutrients and higher in fat, protein and fiber than most other wheats.

Spelt is often used by those dealing with digestive and nervous system disorders, chronic infections, arthritis and cancer, and can substitute for wheat in any bread recipe.

"Develop an attitude toward your bread making and you will feel in harmony with the mysteries of nature and become part of the history of civilization as it is incorporated in each and every loaf of primal bread you bake." Stu Silverstein, Bread on Earth

FERMENTED GRAIN FOODS AND BEVERAGES

Porridge is the mother of us all. (Old Russian proverb)

To prepare an edible grain dish, early peoples generally ground grain and soaked it in water, making a gruel, porridge, or mush which was often then fermented. This fermented porridge was the first widely used grain food. Porridge produced from various grains has been a staple in most parts of the world since prehistory. It is highly likely that experimentation with this staple gruel led to the discovery of leavened bread and beer making.

Fermented gruel is a traditional food of many cultures. The fermentation process, in addition to adding nutritional value, preservatives and natural alcohol to the food, adds flavor to an otherwise monotonous dish. The lactic acid bacteria produce a souring tang, not unlike yogurt or sourdough bread.

Kishk, a fermented wheat porridge made with milk, is a traditional Arab dish that can be stored from winter to summer as a liquid or even longer when dried.

Kaffir beer is a widely consumed beverage made of sorghum and wheat. A pink opaque liquid, the drink has a mealy consistency and a fruit-like tang, and bubbles as it is consumed while still actively fermenting.

Beer is a thin fermented gruel made of mashed, sprouted grain, or malt. When the grain is allowed to sprout, the growing rootlet produces the enzyme *diatase*, which acts on the starch and breaks it down to the simple sugar maltose. During fermentation, yeasts produce alcohol. These yeasts greatly enhance the nutritional properties of the fermenting grains.

Wild yeasts are excellent sources of lysine, riboflavin, niacin and thiamin, and other amino acids and vitamins. Also, the growing yeasts reduce the phytate concentration in grain, improving its digestibility. The yeasts will ferment sugars to alcohol in acidic conditions. The acid conditions of the beer are produced by the fermentation action of lactic acid bacteria, primarily *Lactobacillus, Leuconstococcus, Streptococcus* and *Pediococcus*.

These bacteria add more nutritional value, in the form of protein, amino acids and vitamins, to the food product. Fermented grain foods generally have a protein content 8-20% higher than was originally in the grain. Fermented foods also have enhanced values of thiamine, riboflavin, niacin and amino acids, all vital nutrients for good health.

Fermented foods offer several advantages. The acid conditions produced by the lactic acid bacteria, as well as the alcohol produced by the yeasts, inhibit the growth of putrefying bacteria. Thus the fermenting process acts as a means of preserving food, greatly extending its shelf life. When dried, the fermented food will keep for years, as the low water activity and acid conditions prevent the growth of almost all organisms.

Fermenting is a simple and easy way to enhance the nutritional benefits of our foods and beverages. In places where there is little or no fuel, fermentation offers an additional benefit, in that it requires no heat source, as in cooking or baking.

The earliest evidence of beer consumption comes from a stamp seal found at Tepe Gawra, a Mesopotamian city in northern Iraq. Dated at 4,000 B.C., the stamp shows two figures drinking beer using the traditional straws and container.

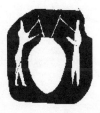

The fermented beverage, about 2% alcohol, was consumed from a clay serving vessel using a large straw made from a reed. Beer was consumed as a food beverage, and a daily ration was approximately 1 liter. Among the Egyptians, beer made from sprouted wheat or barley was an essential ingredient of the daily diet.

Many Sumerian and Mesopotamian texts discuss the preparation and drinking of beer, and these things are depicted in their art. Among the Sumerian texts is found the oldest recorded recipe for beer.

HYMN TO NINKASI.

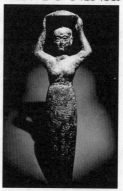

Borne of the flowing water
Tenderly cared for by the Ninhursag
Ninkasi, having founded your town by the sacred lake.
Ninkasi, you are the one who handles the dough
with a big shovel. Mixing in a pit, the bappir with sweet
aromatics and date honey.

Ninkasi, you are the one who bakes
the bappir in the big oven,
Puts in order the piles of hulled grains

Ninkasi, you are the one who waters the malt
set on the ground,
The noble dogs keep away even the potentates.

> Ninkasi, you are the one who soaks
> the malt in a jar.
> The waves rise, the waves fall.
>
> Ninkasi, you are the one who spreads
> the cooked mash on large reed mats.
> Coolness overcomes.
>
> You are the one who holds with both hands
> the great sweet wort. Brewing with honey and wine
>
> You are the sweet wort to the vessel, Ninkasi
> You are the filtering vat, which makes a pleasant sound.
>
> Ninkasi, you are the one who pours out the
> filtered beer of the collector vat,
> It is the onrush of the
> Tigris and Euphrates.

Aside from homemade fermented beverages such as beer, wine and herbal meads, other important fermented foods include all cheeses produced by lactic acid fermentation, yogurt, sauerkraut, kimchee and other fermented vegetables such as pickles, miso and tempeh (both made from fermented soybeans), naturally fermented meats such as sausage, fermented fish and fish sauces, and leavened breads, especially sourdough.

In ancient Rome, sauerkraut was considered delicious and easy to digest and was prized for its medicinal value as well. Large barrels of it were taken on long journeys to the Middle East as the Romans knew it would keep them healthy and protect them from intestinal parasites.

When Pliny wrote in 50 B.C. he described two methods the Italians had for lacto-fermenting cabbage. The first consisted of mashing shredded cabbage in a large earthenware urn which was then hermetically sealed. The second method included mixing vegetables and wild herbs with the cabbage, such as cucumbers, turnips and beets, sorrel and grape leaves, and then covering them with a mixture of water and salt. This method was called a *composituror* mixture. The ancient Greek term for this process was *alchemy*.

Lacto-fermented foods can be eaten as soon as the initial fermentation process is complete. However, these foods improve with age, and experts say it can take up to six months for sauerkraut and other vegetables to fully mature and reach their peak of flavor and nutritional benefits.

Lacto fermenting foods is an artisanal craft. It takes a great deal of time, personal attention to each batch and dedication to perfect the process. Because of this, natural lacto-fermentation does not lend itself to industrialization and these wholesome foods are not readily available to consumers in America.

In the current regulation-crazed social environment of the United States, small scale food production is severely restricted. In most states, dairy farmers cannot sell milk that is not pasteurized and farmers often may not slaughter and process the meat animals they've raised. Homemade breads and fermented food products cannot be sold without a legally certified kitchen.

In his book, *The Revolution Will Not Be Microwaved*, Sandor Ellix Katz laments the fact that *"real, wholesome, local, unadulterated food"* is hard to find in this world of *"dead, processed, industrialized, homogenized, globalized food commodities. Real food is increasingly illegal and being replaced by processed food products. Laws dictating food standards are driven by the model of mass production, where sterility and uniformity are everything, rendering much of the trade in local food technically illegal. Eating well has become an act of civil disobedience."*

My neighbors in the village, where everything is fresh, natural and organic, and an array of lacto-fermented foods are made at home and are commonly available in the local *mercado*, would be very amused by these concepts. Italy is the home of the Slow Food movement, after all. The Italian people are absolutely joyous with food. They take their time growing, gathering, preserving, preparing, serving and consuming it.

In our village the people store much of their garden bounty in little underground rooms, called the *cantina*. One often sees the women and men scurrying from home to their little stone cellar room and carrying back a basket, bottle or armload of stored food or beverage items for dinner.

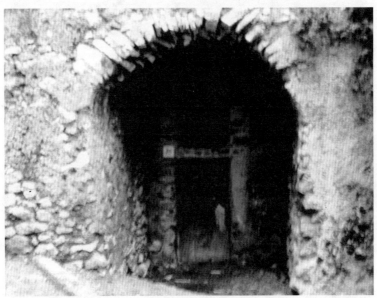

Sitting down to eat a meal together is something the people here do every day. Around 1:30 in the afternoon one hears pots, pans and dishes rattling in the nearby homes and the sounds of people serving and eating food, talking and laughing. Eating is an enjoyable social occasion here and goes on for quite a while.

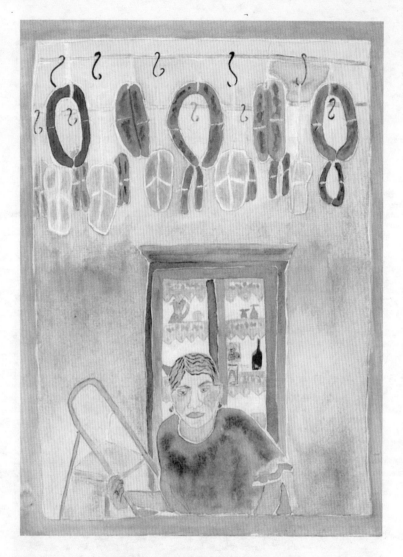

My *vacina* (neighbor) Rosina, and her daughter Maria, are masters of sausage making. In December they slaughter their pigs and make several different kinds of sausage, like many others in the village. They then hang each one from a hook attached to long poles suspended from Rosina's kitchen ceiling. The heat from the fireplace slowly cures the sausage over the following months.

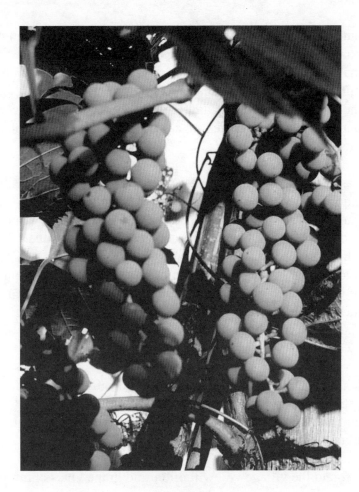

Grapes
Vitis vinifera
V. labrusca and V. rotundifolia

"I am the vine and you are the branches." John 15:3

Over the many years that I have lived on our herb farm in Maine, I have discovered that grapes are a lot of fun. There is no other way to put it. I've always loved gathering baskets full of wild grapes in late summer from the hedgerows, where they thrive with wild abandon all around our farm. Some years these wild vines offer a profusion of bunches of small purple grapes, a bit tart, but perfect for making wine. I often gather and dry grape leaves for mineral rich teas, and usually wrap the vines, after stripping the leaves, into wreaths and crowns. In recent years we've planted several varieties of cultivated grape vines around the gardens.

Last year was the first time I pruned these grapes. I really enjoyed the task. Grape vines are simply magical. The gardeners among us know that so much about gardening, and tending plants, can be compared with spiritual life. Clippers in hand, I spent what turned out to be most of the afternoon climbing around the grape arbors, rolling around on my knees, stretching up as high as I could reach on my toes, pruning away errant new growth down to two main leaders. Every branch I trimmed, another shortcoming fell away.

I have watched the old people around our village in Italy pruning their grape vines. I tried to give my work the love and attention I have seen on their faces and in their hands. I know I could feel it in my heart.

Around the village you will often find grape vines climbing up trellises that are built at the entrance to the home, each one a unique and beautifully pruned masterpiece. And where there is a lack of space you will find vines growing out of big ceramic urns, tumbling off of terraces, and next to Carmella's *casa* there is a thick, ancient grape vine sticking out of a space between the cobblestone and the house!

The Mediterranean peoples all love grapes and have been using the fruits of this vine, and the wine they make from it, for therapeutic value since time immemorial. They know that fermented drinks like natural organic grape wine and herbal meads are health-promoting, and especially nourishing to the brain, heart, circulatory system and liver.

Drinking a small glass of home-made grape wine regularly, as most Mediterranean people do at dinner, helps to keep the heart functioning well into old age, keeps cholesterol as well as blood pressure down, and invigorates the brain and all body systems.

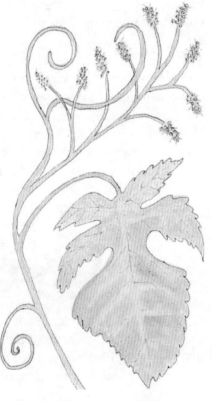

Of course, grapes themselves are a supreme and delicious food and medicine. Grapes strengthen and restore the entire body, and all parts of the grape plant, leaves, tendrils, stem and fruit, offer abundant iron, calcium, potassium, as well as a wealth of other health and vitality boosting nutrients.

In fact, the ability of grapes to alleviate fatigue is astonishing. Grape sugars are different from other sugars. They are absorbed into the blood stream much more rapidly, go to work quickly, and bring both strength and tone to the entire body. For this reason, I prefer to use distilled grape alcohol for the tinctures I make. I have found them to be not only superior in taste, but also in effectiveness.

Grapes and grape juice, fermented or not, act as a warming tonic to the digestive system, benefit the kidneys and promote a free flow of urine. Grapes not only offer invigoration and vitality, but fertility as well.

Grapes, as well as the leaves and tendrils, are highly regarded as fertility enhancers. I've used them for many years in combination with red clover and red raspberry leaves, and have seen many babies born after their mothers consumed this simple formula.

The latest scientific research is suggesting that long-lived and nourishing grape vines may also help prolong our lives by protecting our cells against aging. Resveratrol, a natural compound found in grapes (and also in mulberries, peanuts, blueberries, bilberries, cranberries, some pines, and the roots of Japanese knotweed) appears to protect against cancer, cardiovascular and other diseases by acting as an antioxidant, antimutagen, antiviral, neuroprotective and anti-inflammatory agent.

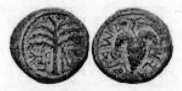

Resveratrol is also under extensive investigation as a cancer preventive agent. Recently published studies have shown that resveratrol interferes with and inhibits all three stages of carcinogenesis - initiation, promotion and progression.

Moderate wine consumption may help protect against Alzheimer's disease. Population studies indicate a link between moderate consumption of red wine and a lower incidence of Alzheimer's disease. A laboratory study published in the *Journal of Biological Chemistry* helps explain why. Resveratrol greatly reduces the levels of amyloid-beta peptides (Abeta). Plaques containing Abeta are a hallmark in the brain tissue of patients with Alzheimer's disease.

Grape seeds are good for us also! Vitamin E, flavonoids, linoleic acid, and compounds called procyanidins (also known as pycnogenols, and oligomeric proanthocyanidins or OPCs) are highly concentrated in grape seeds. These healthful compounds can also be found in lower concentrations in the skin of the grape.

Proanthocyanidic acid is a powerful antioxidant and anti-inflammatory agent that can reduce the damage done by free radicals, strengthen and repair connective tissue, and promote enzyme activity. It also helps moderate allergic and inflammatory responses by reducing histamine production.

There are two main species of grapes:

EUROPEAN GRAPES (*Vitis vinifera*): These include Thompson (seedless and amber-green in color), Emperor (seeded and purple in color) and Champagne/Black Corinth (tiny in size and purple in color). European varieties feature skins that adhere closely to their flesh.

NORTH AMERICAN GRAPES (*Vitis labrusca* and *Vitis rotundifolia*): Varieties include Concord (blue-black in color and large in size), Delaware (pink-red in color with a tender skin) and Niagara (amber colored and less sweet than other varieties). North American varieties feature skins that more easily slip away from their flesh.

No matter if you have a nice sized garden plot, or just a five-gallon pail near a window, I encourage you to try growing a nourishing, magical, healing grape vine. Your health may improve, you'll have more fun, and your life might last longer too!

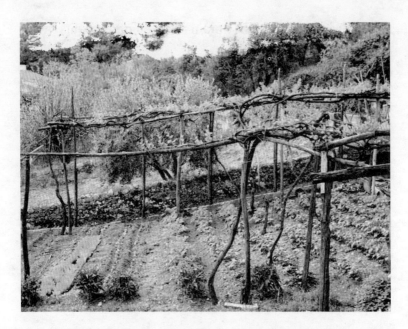

MY VISITS WITH FRANCESCA

Francesca is 78 years old, a widow for the past nine years, and the sister of my neighbor, Carmella, with whom I share this lovely little courtyard. Francesca and I met the first year I came to Monte San Giacomo, as she lived next door to the house where my grandmothers were born and raised, and my daughters and I were fortunate to have stayed on our first visit here just a few years ago. I've been visiting regularly with Francesca ever since, during the winter months that I spend here in the village.

That first year Francesca would come over every morning for a visit around 9AM towing along her little grandson, Fabio, then about three years old. Fabio was so cute, so full of energy and loved to play soccer in the kitchen of my grandmother's house. He also loved to *"scriva"* (write), so we would give him a pencil and paper, sit him at the table and he would happily alternate between these two activities for the hour or so that Francesca sat in the kitchen talking non-stop to me in rapid fire San Giacomese dialect.

You see, here in Southern Italia, every village has its own dialect. People in one village can sometimes barely understand the dialect of people in the next village over. Italy has been working to remedy this situation since the unification of the country, teaching the common Italian language in all the schools in hopes of creating one Italian language. Meanwhile, the old people like Francesca continue speaking the only language they know, their local dialect.

All of the children here are bilingual – they are fluent in both the dialect, which they speak at home and to each other, and the common Italian, which they speak formally.

Now Francesca, like many Italians, is exceptionally expressive and animated. During our visits she waves her arms freely about her, uses a multitude of vivid hand signals as she speaks, and changes her facial expression moment to moment, as well as the tone of her voice. Though I do not know most of the words she speaks, it is not difficult to get the overall meaning of what she is saying. She laughs, she sighs, and she smiles, she whines and cries, and in short, articulates a wider range of emotions in one paragraph than most Americans do in a month!

So we sit together in front of the fireplace in my kitchen some mornings, talking and enjoying the warmth of the fire. She is inevitably dressed from head to toe in black. Today, as usual, she is wearing a black dress and a button down sweater with two pockets, one of which always contains her house keys. She has her black stockings rolled up just over her knees and wears a pair of walking slippers on her swollen feet. Her thick grey hair is fixed into a bun at the back of her head, and loose wisps of it fly about her head as she speaks.

Since she lived next door to my ancestral home for most of her life, she knows my family very well. My great-uncle, Zimmatteo, the brother of my grandmother, Maria Giuseppa, lived in that house after my grandmother left for America, and raised his eight children there. Zimmatteo, as he is referred to by all, is a much loved figure in our village, well remembered by all the older people here. Among many other things, he contributed very generously to the Church of Sant Antonio. Evidently, Sant Antonio, who is the protector of orphaned children, was a great inspiration for my uncle Zimmatteo. His first wife died, leaving him with three young children to care for. He married a second wife, who shortly after passed away, and then a third, with whom he finally shared a long and prosperous life, and who bore him five more children. One of those daughters, Angelina, took over our family home, and her descendents live there now.

So Francesca knows all the family stories, from way back, and tells them to me in these morning visits. How I wish I clearly understood every word she speaks, as she is a brilliant story teller, who spins vividly emotional and colorful tales. And these family tales, I realize, will mostly disappear with her. So I listen intently, with full attention, as she speaks. I am completely focused on absorbing these stories, and they take on new life as she recounts them, and I hear them in my own way. Someday I will be passing along these same stories, to another generation eager to learn who they are and where they come from. You see, I decided right away to be the keeper of Francesca's tales. And since my understanding of the dialect is extremely limited, I do not know exactly whose family member had their hand caught in a car door and had to go to the hospital, or who it was that was throwing up all night in the bathroom just before they died. Francesca not only speaks non-stop, and rapid fire, but jumps from topic to topic, family to family, making it next to impossible for me to keep all the stories straight. No matter. I sit there in the kitchen by the fire, patiently nodding my head, changing my facial expressions along with hers, saying *oh no, ah peccato!,* or *si, si, si,* as seems appropriate.

After about an hour my head is spinning and my neck hurts. I cannot absorb a single phrase more. I realize as each visit goes by, though, that I recognize a little more of the pattern and rhythm of her lyric speech, and single words have begun to be clear to me. She's been teaching me! My understanding of our native dialect is growing by the half inch daily, but still, it is progress. *Poco, poco,* little by little, as they are fond of saying here. What I have learned most of all from these mornings with Francesca is that often times words are irrelevant. Body language, tone of voice, facial expressions, and hand signals - these are the true and universal modes of communication.

Francesca senses that our visit is coming to an end and begins to make moves to depart. She wraps her sweater up around her ample breasts, jingles the keys in her pocket, moves her feet from side to side. She has a few more things to say, and does so freely, then gets up from her chair by the fire. I rise too, and together we walk over to the door. We kiss each other on both cheeks, and then hug each other tightly. I love this aged woman who carries so much of my family history, all these old memories, and so much love in her heart.

My love is spilling over on her now as she hobbles on her hurt feet out of the door and I cannot resist patting her gently once more on her back as she heads down the steps. I say to her, "*Grazie* for coming today Francesca, I love our visits, come again soon," in English, and she turns around beaming at me, and I understand that for her too our visits are about much more than mere words.

Francesca heads around the corner and down the ramp into her sister Carmella's garden, and disappears between rows of mustard and 4-foot-high broccolini. She'll be bringing a big bag of these flower heads back home with her. Carmella usually harvests all she can every day from the long rows they have back there, and often brings some over for me. What a delicious and nourishing treat!

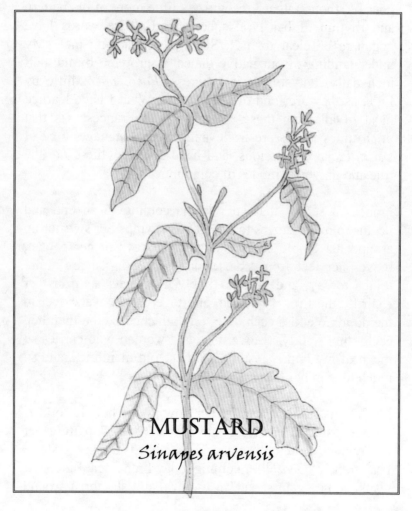

MUSTARD
Sinapes arvensis

MUSTARD, CABBAGE, BROCCOLI
Brassicaceae Family

formerly Cruciferous, aka *The Cabbage Family*

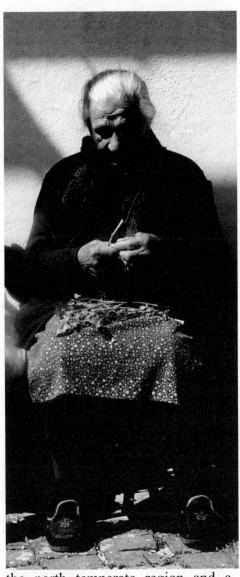

This is a large family with many tasty, nourishing and useful plants, including a few well known and familiar vegetables (cabbage, turnip), oil crops (rape), medicinal herbs (shepherd's purse), and ornamentals (alyssum).

They are found all over the world, with many of the species occurring in the north temperate region and a few in the southern hemisphere.

They are mostly annual or perennial herbaceous plants, with one or two small shrubs or climbers.

CHARACTERISTICS:

LEAVES, STEM AND ROOTS The leaves are usually alternate up the stem. Edible species have been selected and bred to maximize the size of the part used - large, fleshy roots as in turnips, large leaves as in cabbages, large flower buds as in cauliflower and broccoli.

FLOWERS The flowers give this plant family its original name of Cruciferae. They are cruciform, made up of four petals in the shape of a cross. They are usually in clusters or heads, and the flowers are usually white or yellow, although they may be an array of colors when cultivated for ornamental use.

SEEDS The seed pods of this plant family are also easily identifiable. They are formed of two chambers joined by a thin membrane, which opens from the bottom. The flat membrane often remains after the outer surface of the seed capsule has been shed.

The cabbage family plants provide us with a great diversity of both nutrients and flavors. You might consider that a daily bowl of any of these greens or roots is indispensable for good health: radish, turnips, shepherd's purse, bok choi, napa, Chinese cabbage, broccoli rabe, kohlrabi, mustard greens, kale, broccoli, cauliflower, Brussels sprouts, cabbage and cress.

In the village even the simplest meal usually includes several courses. One of those courses is always freshly cooked greens. These are very hardy plants, and can usually withstand cool temperatures. In southern Italy they are grown during the winter months. A short row of any of these plants will yield enough greens for a meal every day.

radish, turnips, shepherds purse,
bok choi, napa, Chinese cabbage,
broccoli rabe, kohlrabi, mustard greens,
kale, broccoli, cauliflower, brussels sprouts,
cabbage and cress.

BROCCOLI *Brassica oleracea* (botrytis group)
cultivation originated in Italy.

Broccolo, as it is known in Italian, means "cabbage sprout." The ancient Romans were inspired horticulturists and developed broccoli from their wild cabbage. Broccoli's name is derived from the Latin word *brachium*, which means branch or arm, and describes its growing appearance.

One of the most popular types of broccoli sold in North America is known as Italian green, or Calabrese, named after the Italian province of Calabria where it was first grown. Broccoli was introduced to the United States in colonial times and popularized by Italian immigrants who brought this prized vegetable with them to the New World.

Members of the *Brassica* family offer uniquely important health-promoting properties. In addition to the wide array of necessary vitamins and minerals they provide, *Brassica* vegetables also contain a number of especially potent health enhancing and protective phytonutrients.

For instance, certain compounds in these vegetables known as *glucosinolates* react with an enzyme called *myrosinase* that converts them into *indoles* and *isothiocyanates*. *Indoles* and *isothiocyanates* reduce the potential of carcinogens through their ability to stimulate liver detoxification enzymes. These phytonutrients inhibit certain enzymes that normally activate carcinogens and also induce other enzymes that help to dismantle active carcinogens.

Sulforaphane, another interesting compound found in the vegetables in this family, is actually formed when cruciferous vegetables such as mustard greens and broccoli are chopped or chewed. It, too, is known to trigger the liver to produce enzymes that detoxify cancer-causing chemicals. Sulforaphane has been shown to inhibit chemically-induced breast cancers, reverse colon cancer cells and stop the proliferation of breast cancer cells, even in the later stages of their growth.

When scientists at the World Cancer Research Fund reviewed 206 human and 22 animal studies, they reported finding convincing evidence that cruciferous vegetables provide excellent protection against many forms of cancer, including tumors of the stomach, pancreas, esophagus, lung, oral cavity and pharynx, endometrium, breast, ovaries, prostate and colon.

Now, research published in the *International Journal of Cancer* (Zhao, H. Lin, J.) suggests that bladder cancer can join the list. Those in the study eating the most cruciferous vegetables were found to have a 29% lower risk of bladder cancer compared to participants eating the least amount of this family of vegetables.

How many weekly servings of Brassicas do we need to protect against cancer? Just 3 to 5 servings per week, less than one serving a day! (1 serving = 1 cup)

Consider sprouting broccoli seeds and eating the sprouts. They are exceptionally rich in sulforaphane, 10 to 100 times as rich as the mature broccoli.

Other constituents of note include lutein, a form of the antioxidant vitamin A, found to offer considerable protection against the formation of cataracts. Still other compounds in these vegetables offer protection against heart disease and stroke, act to prevent skin cell changes due to sun exposure, inhibit the growth of *H. pylori* (which causes ulcers) in the gut, and serve as supreme immune system nourishers. The calcium-rich vegetables in this family also help to build strong bones, teeth, hair and nails.

One cup of cooked broccoli contains 74 mg of calcium, plus 123 mg of vitamin C, which significantly improves the absorption of calcium. It also offers 1359 mcg of beta-carotene, and useful amounts of zinc and selenium, trace minerals that play vital roles in immune system health. A cup of broccoli has 44 calories and supplies 94 mcg of folic acid, a critically important B vitamin especially necessary during pregnancy to ensure a healthy fetus.

A study published in the *Journal of the Science of Food and Agriculture* investigated the effects of various methods of cooking broccoli. Of all the methods of preparation, steaming caused the least loss of nutrients. Microwaving broccoli resulted in a loss of 97% to 74% of the major antioxidant compounds, flavonoids. In comparison, steaming broccoli resulted in a loss of only 11% to 8% of the same antioxidants.

Study co-author Dr. Cristina Garcia-Viguera noted that *"Most of the bioactive compounds are water-soluble; during heating, they leach in a high percentage into the cooking water. Because of this, it is recommended to cook vegetables in the minimum amount of water (as in steaming) in order to retain their nutritional benefits."*

In addition to enhancing bone health, the nutrients in Brassicas can help ease our way through menopause. The abundant levels of magnesium are exceedingly nourishing to the nervous system and have proven helpful in reducing anxiety and stress as well as promoting healthy sleeping patterns. Vitamin E, also found in plentiful amounts in these foods, has also been shown to decrease the occurrence and severity of hot flashes.

Caution: Brassicas contain goitrogens, naturally-occurring substances in certain foods that can interfere with the function of the thyroid gland. Individuals with existing and untreated thyroid problems may want to avoid broccoli and other foods in this group. Cooking may help to inactivate the goitrogenic compounds found in these foods, but it isn't clear just how many of them are affected or how much.

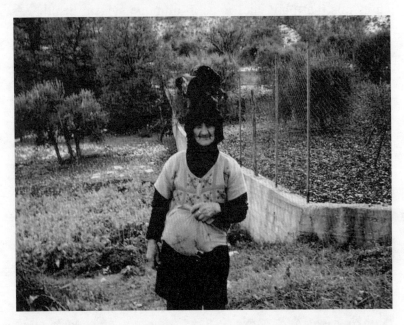

MUSTARD GREENS Sinapes arvensis posses a sharp, peppery flavor, add zest and lots of nourishment to any meal and are at their peak during the winter months in Southern Italy. See the patch of mustard greens in the background of the picture above? This beautiful woman has a shirt full of the greens she has just harvested. In a moment she will give them all to my daughter Grace, who is taking the picture, insisting that she take them home with her to share with our family. All the while balancing that large chunk of wood she is carrying on her head!

Mustard greens are the leaves of the mustard plant, *Brassica juncea*. The greens can have either a crumpled or flat texture and may have toothed, scalloped, frilled or lacey edges. There are lots of varieties of mustard and each has distinct characteristics. Most mustard greens are an emerald green color but they can also be shades of dark red or deep purple.

In addition to its nutritious greens, this plant also produces the acrid-tasting brown seeds that are used to make Dijon mustard.

Mustard greens originated in the Himalayan region of India and have been grown and consumed for more than 5,000 years. They are a notable vegetable in many different cuisines, including Italian, Chinese and Southern American. Like turnip greens, mustard greens became an integral part of Southern cuisine during the times of slavery.

Mustard greens are an excellent source of many vitamins, including vitamin A, vitamin C, folate and vitamin E. They also offer an excellent source of the mineral manganese and plenty of B6, calcium and copper. They are also a very good source of phosphorus, vitamins B1 and B2, magnesium, protein, potassium and iron. Mustard greens provide fiber, are low in calories and high in antioxidants.

Studies have shown that mustard greens share the anticancer effects of the other Brassicas. They have the ability to protect against breast cancer and heart disease. Their high content of nutrients (such as calcium, folic acid and magnesium) also supports strong healthy bones.

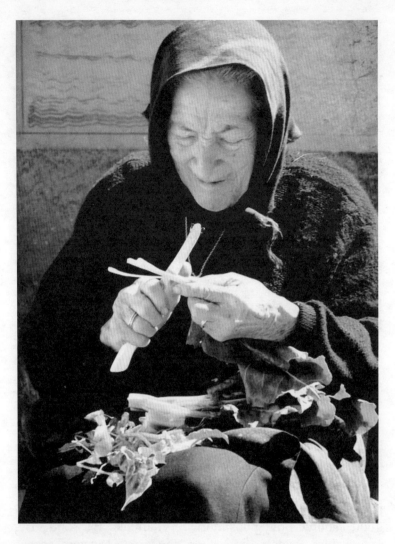

ASPARAGUS *Asparagus officinalis* is low in calories and carbohydrates, and compared to other vegetables, relatively high in protein. One cup of asparagus supplies only 24 calories, almost half of which are derived from protein. Asparagus is an excellent source of potassium, vitamin K, folic acid (263 mcg per cup), vitamins C and A, riboflavin, thiamine, and vitamin B6.

Asparagus is also a very good source of dietary fiber, niacin, phosphorus and iron.

In early spring we climb the mountainsides along with many others from our village, hunting for and gathering wild asparagus shoots. They are quite a bit smaller than the cultivated variety, but oh, so delicious!

Historically, asparagus has been used as a diuretic and for the management of arthritis and rheumatism. The amino acid *asparagine* may be responsible for the diuretic effect of asparagus. When this amino acid is excreted in the urine, it gives off a strong, characteristic odor.

CABBAGE *Brassica oleracea* (capitata group) is

another low calorie, nutrient-dense food that offers an excellent source of many nutrients, including vitamin C, folic acid, potassium, vitamin B6, calcium, biotin, magnesium and manganese. Along with its nutrient content, cabbage also contains the powerful anticancer compounds known as glucosinolates.

One of the dietary recommendations from the American Cancer Society is to regularly include cruciferous vegetables such as mustard, cabbage, Brussels sprouts, broccoli, and cauliflower in the diet.

The glucosinolates in these plants function by increasing the antioxidant defense mechanisms and by improving the body's ability to detoxify and eliminate harmful chemicals and hormones. Studies have shown that cabbage is also extremely effective in the treatment of peptic ulcers.

CAULIFLOWER *Brassica oleracea* (botrytis group)

is not as nutrient-dense as many of the other vegetables in the cabbage family, but is an excellent source of vitamins C and K. It is also a very good source of potassium, fiber, phosphorus and B vitamins and offers the trace mineral boron. Like other members of the family, it contains several cancer fighting phytochemicals in the form of glucosinolates

BRUSSELS SPROUTS *Brassica oleracea*

(gemmifera group) have similar nutritional qualities as broccoli. They are a great source of folic acid, vitamins C and K, and beta carotene. They provide plenty of vitamin B6, fiber, thiamine, potassium and those all-important cancer-fighting glucosinolates.

KALE is an excellent source of vitamins B6 and C, carotenes and manganese. It's a good source of vitamins B1, B2 and E, fiber, iron, copper, calcium and phosphorus. Kale and collard greens exhibit the same anticancer properties as other members of the cabbage family.

RADISHES *Raphanus sativus* and their greens provide an excellent source of vitamin C. Radish leaves contain almost six times as much vitamin C as their roots and are a good source of calcium and protein. Daikon radishes provide a very good source of potassium and copper. Like other members of this plant family, they also contain cancer-protective properties. Radishes have a strong reputation and history of being used as medicine for liver disorders. They contain a variety of sulfur-based chemicals that increase the flow of bile. Therefore, radishes in the diet help to maintain a healthy gall bladder and liver, and will improve digestion. Fresh radish roots contain a larger amount of vitamin C than cooked radish roots.

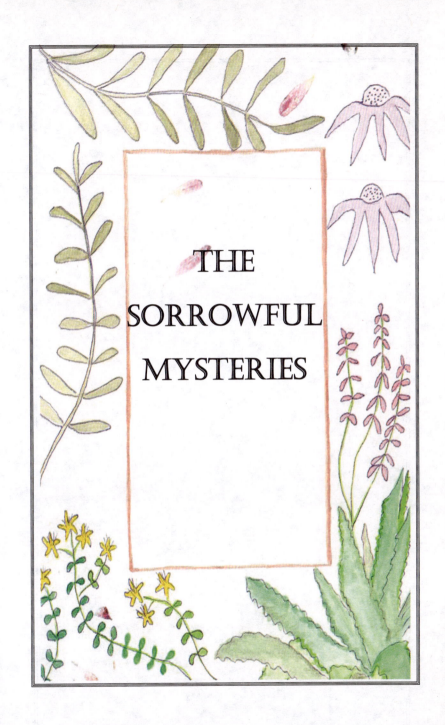

THE SORROWFUL MYSTERIES

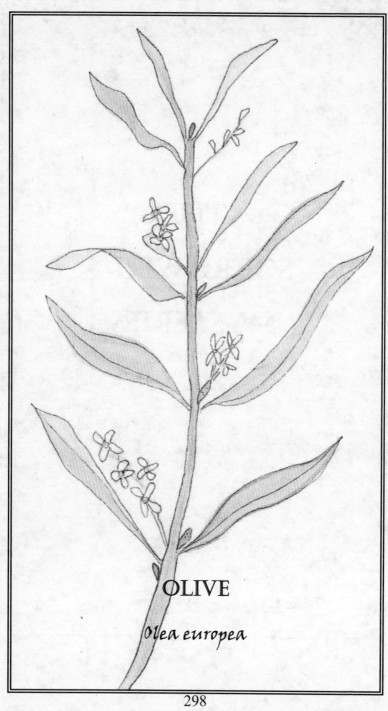

SORROWFUL MYSTERIES

The Sorrowful Mysteries bring awareness to the Olive Tree, St. John's wort, Aloe vera and passionflower.

SEAT OF WISDOM –THE OLIVE TREE

Among the most beautiful and inspiring sights in all of Italy are the gorgeous grey-green olive tree groves.

Wherever you drive along the Amalfi coast, across inland valleys, or head south through the mountains to the sea, you'll sees well tended olive trees being cultivated in long neat rows, climbing up the hillsides in all directions. Often while walking around the edges of our village where all the gardens are planted and our local olive trees grow, we come upon an old man or woman, up in his or her olive tree, happily pruning back the thorny branches.

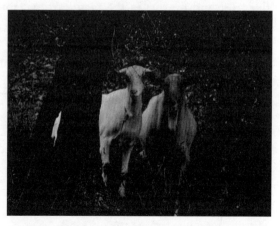

One glorious bright winter day my three daughters and I had the great pleasure of helping our friend Angela harvest some of her olives. While her goats grazed nearby, strong, sturdy, vibrant Angela, in her mid-seventies, easily hauled a ladder to each tree, climbed up into it and shook the branches until a shower of olives rained down onto a plastic sheet we'd placed underneath. Our job was to filter out the leaves and scoop the olives up into clean while pails.

When the pails were full, Angela emptied the olives into a large burlap bag, placed it on her head and waved good-bye to us. She turned around and began chasing her goats up the hill, waving her arms up over her head and shouting at them, all the while balancing that huge bag of olives on her head. Then, half-way up the hill, as we watched in utter amazement, Angela bent over to grab a large piece of fire wood, slung it over her left shoulder, and without missing a beat, kept running behind the goats, the burlap bag full of olives still poised gracefully on her head...

What is in these olives, I wondered, that helps to keep the old people here, like Angela, so youthful, healthy, happy and vibrant? I'd like to share with you what I found.

Olives, a staple food of the Mediterranean diet, are fruits of the tree known as *Olea europea*. "Olea" is the Latin word for "oil" and describes the natural juice that is pressed from the fruit and preserves the taste, aroma, vitamins and other nourishing properties of the olive. Olive oil is the only vegetable oil that can be consumed as it is - freshly pressed from the fruit, requiring no further processing.

Olive trees are extremely long-lived, with many living longer than a thousand years. A small evergreen, the olive tree matures between 50 and 100 years of age. The tree bears small, fragrant, creamy white flowers in May, and its leaves are pale green above and silvery below. Its fruit is ready to harvest from November through January.

Originating from the Mesopotamia, the olive was spread by the Phoenicians and grows almost exclusively around the Mediterranean. It is found in calcareous hilly terrain and is quite resistant to dryness and to infertile soils. In fact the olive tree is said to grow even from bare rocks and requires very little water. It has long been a symbol of endurance.

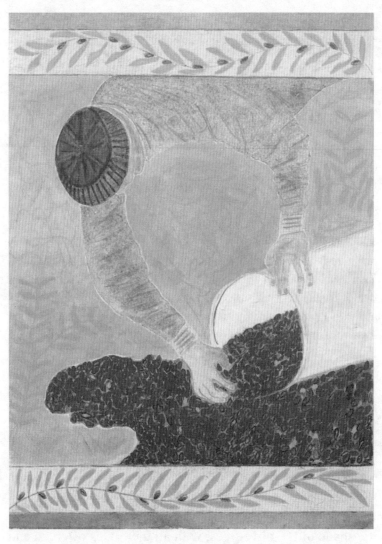

Olives, one of the oldest foods known, are mentioned often in the Bible and depicted in ancient Egyptian art, and played an important role in Greek mythology. Hippocrates, often referred to as the father of medicine, called olives and their oil "the great therapeutic."

Since ancient times, the olive tree has provided food, fuel, timber and medicine for many civilizations. Olive oil has been consumed since at least 3,000 B.C. It has long been regarded as a symbol of peace and wisdom.

The Blessed Mother has been referred to by such names as *The Fruitful Olive Tree, God's Olive Tree* and *"Fair olive tree of the plains."*

Muhammad tells us to use olive oil and anoint yourself with it, because it is "from a blessed tree." Ancient Greek legends tell of the creation of the olive tree by the goddess Athena, who also taught the people its many healing uses.

The Midrash teaches that the branch carried back to Noah's ark after the flood, marking the "renewal of life," was taken from the slopes of the Mount of Olives. Of all the hills in the Jerusalem area, the Mount of Olives is the tallest - about 830 meters high at its peak and from the top, one has a panoramic view of the old and new cities of Jerusalem on the west and the Judean Desert on the east.

According to tradition, the royal graves of some of the kings of the House of David, and particularly that of King Uzziah, may have been nearby. This then was the burial ground of Jesus' ancestors. It was sacred ground.

The Garden of Gethsemane, which means *the garden with the olive press*, lies at the foot of the Mount of Olives and was a favorite place of Jesus. He must have liked it there in the shade of the olive trees, with all their hues of green and silver, casting light about like spirit dancing on the breeze. He often gathered followers and shared his teachings on this hallowed ground, and it was to this garden that Jesus went to pray, and from where he was taken after the Last Supper, and the place from which he is said to have ascended into heaven. This sacred olive grove is the scene of many poignant and significant New Testament scenes.

Olives have a long association with the sacred. Its oil has been used to anoint sacred objects, places and people for many thousands of years. Olives have also produced the oil used in cooking, preserving, healing and beautifying, as well as for ceremony and blessings throughout millennia. The New Testament tells us of many who were sick and anointed with oil and made well again. Ancient surgeons used olive leaves to make plasters and the oil was used in liniments for treating wounds and skin afflictions.

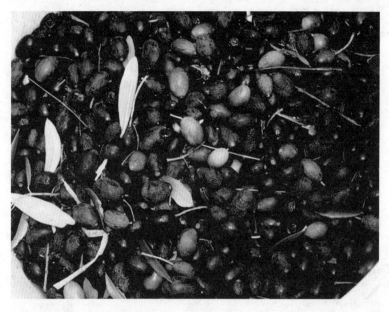

Olive oil is very high in fat content (15-35%) of which 75% is oleic acid, a monounsaturated fat known to lower blood cholesterol levels, as well as high blood pressure.

A study in the March 27, 2000 issue of the journal *Archives of Internal Medicine* reports that people on high blood pressure medications may be able to reduce the amount of medicine they take if they substitute extra-virgin olive oil for other fats in their diet. "The most important finding in this study is that the daily use of olive oil, about 40 grams per day (equal to four tablespoons), markedly reduces the dosage of blood pressure medication by about 50% in hypertensive patients on a previously stable drug dosage," says L. Aldo Ferrara, MD, associate professor of internal medicine at the Frederico II University of Naples in Naples, Italy, and the study's author.

Olives are not only an excellent source of monounsaturated fats, but also offer an abundance of vitamin E, and so protect our cells from free radicals, lowering the risk of both cellular damage and inflammation. For example, when free radicals cause the oxidation of cholesterol, the oxidized cholesterol damages blood vessels and builds up in the arteries, which can eventually lead to heart attack or stroke. By preventing the oxidation of cholesterol, the nutrients in olives help protect the heart, preventing heart disease as well as stroke.

Beneficial phytonutrients such as polyphenols and flavonoids, appear to have strong anti-inflammatory properties and may help reduce the severity of asthma, osteoarthritis and rheumatoid arthritis.

A higher intake of both the vitamin E and the monounsaturated fats available in olives is also associated with lower rates of colon cancer. In fact, a recently published study by researchers at the University of Oxford adds to the growing body of evidence that shows olive oil is as good as fresh fruit and vegetables in keeping colon cancer at bay.

Dr. Michael Goldacre and researchers at the Institute of Health Sciences compared cancer rates, diets and olive oil consumption in 28 countries, including Europe, Britain, the United States, Brazil, Colombia, Canada and China. Countries with a diet high in meat and low in vegetables had the highest rates of cancer, and olive oil was associated with decreased risk.

The researchers suspect olive oil protects against bowel cancer by influencing the metabolism of the digestive system. "Olive oil seems to reduce the amount of bile acid and increase the levels of the enzyme thought to beneficially regulate cell turnover in the gut," Goldacre said.

With its ability to slow down acid overproduction in the digestive system, olive oil also diminishes the potential for ulcers and other gastrointestinal problems.

Of course, all traditionally lacto-fermented foods including olives, pickles, cheese, wine, mead, yogurt, sauerkraut and sausages, offer wonderful benefits for the digestive system. In fact, these naturally fermented foods and beverages are now considered to be "probiotics," promoting the growth of friendly intestinal bacteria, aiding digestion and supporting immune function. Furthermore, the nutrients available in these foods, such as B vitamins (including vitamin B12), omega-3 fatty acids, digestive enzymes, lactase and lactic acid, and other nutrients, are actually increased by fermentation.

SKIN & BEAUTY CARE
Studies have clearly shown the benefits of olive oil over safflower and fish oil on pre-cancerous cells. Japanese scientists claim that extra virgin olive oil applied to the skin after sunbathing could protect against skin cancer by slowing tumor growth.

Olive oil has long been a treasured beauty secret in Italy. For centuries, women in the Mediterranean area have been using olive products to enhance their beauty, invigorate their souls and ensure good health. The antioxidant vitamins E and A have been proven to be very helpful against sun damage. Vitamin E, a powerful antioxidant with skin protective and moisturizing properties, prevents skin irritation and premature aging of the skin. It also offers anti-inflammatory properties. Vitamin A is another potent antioxidant with skin regenerative properties. It helps the skin stay soft, smooth and firm, increases elasticity and has anti-aging benefits.

It's been found that olive oil softens and hydrates without blocking the natural function of the skin. My beautiful Italian mother told me long ago that to improve skin tone and prevent wrinkles, be sure to have two or three tablespoons of olive oil in the daily diet. Ancient legends say that "olive oil makes aches and pains go away."

When making herbal infused oils to apply to the skin, I prefer to use pure olive oil. It has been the extractor and fixative of choice for herbalists down through the centuries. Olive oil is great for relaxing massages and is perfect for sensitive skin. It's been found that Greek women, who use plenty of olive products in their diets, have a 42% lower rate of breast cancer than women in the United States.

Olive is an important food ingredient no matter what your age. Olive oil is recognized as important in maintaining metabolism and contributes to the development of the brain and bones in children. And, it is recommended as a source of vitamin E for older people. With its rich supply of natural anti-oxidants, olive oil considerably slows down the aging process.

When buying olive oil for food consumption, look for quality EXTRA VIRGIN oil. The oil that comes from the first "pressing" of the olive, is extracted without using heat (a cold press) or chemicals, and has no "off" flavors is awarded "extra virgin" status. Keep olive oil in a cool and dark place, tightly sealed. Oxygen promotes rancidity.

ST. JOHN'S WORT
Hypericum perforatum

Mary was perceived, in accordance with the prophecy of Simeon, as sharing directly in Christ's suffering both spiritually and emotionally. The sword of sorrow was to pierce her heart also.

St. John's wort speaks to us of the Sorrowful Mother aspect of Mary. On Good Friday evening it is this Sorrowful Mother who is carried through the streets of my village, while the parishioners wail an ancient and mournful dirge in the torch-lit procession that trails behind her.

This perception of Mary as having suffered along with Jesus and the association of this facet of the story with St. John's wort is acknowledged by the Gaelic peoples, among whom St. John's wort is called *Allus Muire* or Mary's Sweat. In other areas this plant is known as Christ's Sweat and sometimes Christ's Blood.

These associations relate to the tiny red dots, or oil glands, that can be seen on the leaves and blooms of St. John's wort. These glands hold a red ink-like substance, called *hypericin,* which oozes from the flower bud when squeezed between the fingers.

This hypericin, as well as several other constituents of St. John's wort, has strong and impressive anti-inflammatory actions and pain relieving qualities. Additionally, St. John's wort is a highly respected nerve restorative, and will heal and actually rejuvenate damaged nerves.

This plant is known and respected the world over for its capacity to offer comfort and solace, for its ability to lift, enhance and protect the human spirit. St. John's wort has ancient associations with the sacred that far predate Christianity, Jesus and Mary.

Since the earliest times it has been associated with spiritual protection and magic. The ancients used it as a fumigant, a cleanser. St. John's wort has been burned and otherwise used for the purpose of ridding "evil spirits" from a person or place since time immemorial. This particular herb was, and may still be, used by the Catholic Church in exorcisms, which still do, though rarely, occur. Such is the long-time reputation of this profoundly sacred and potent herb.

During the Middle Ages flowers with potent medicinal qualities were often named after the saints whose feast days were celebrated at the time of their bloom. Thus this plant, which blooms in mid-June in European countries, became associated with St. John the Baptist, whose feast is celebrated at the summer solstice and who represents the strong ascending power of the sun.

In Italy, where this herb is referred to as *Herba Sant Giovanni,* it is soaked in olive oil for several weeks, strained, and then the oil is used to ease aches and pains, or as a "balm for every wound." It may also serve as a sacred oil, perhaps for private prayer or the consecration of a sacred object.

In the same way that St. John's wort is respected for ensuring no harm comes to the human spirit, so it also protects the physical body from invading, disease-causing organisms. This herb's antiviral, antibacterial and antifungal effects are legendary. It seems to create an impenetrable shield, preventing disease from gaining a foothold and supporting strong immunity, thus protecting from within.

ALOE VERA
Aloe Barbadensis Miller

The word Aloe in Sanskrit means Goddess.

Aloe vera and related species are known by such names as healing plant, miracle plant, burn plant, first aid plant, lily of the desert, jelly leek, plant of life and plant of immortality.

Originally a native of South and East Africa, this remarkable plant has spread all over the world. Flourishing in warm, dry climates, it is cultivated in tropical and subtropical regions and grows abundantly throughout the Mediterranean area.

A member of the Liliacea family, it is a succulent perennial, grows in a clump and has long, spiky, grey-green leaves. There are approximately 400 species of Aloe, but it is the *Aloe Barbadensis Miller*, or "true aloe," referred to as Aloe vera, that possesses the most remarkable healing properties. Aloe vera has an ancient association with the sacred Trinity, as the foliage emerges from the base of the plant in groups of three.

I've seen many humongous Aloe vera plants rising up from the mountainsides throughout Southern Italy, as well as in and around people's gardens. The plant is widely used and respected by the people here. Home in Maine, we grow Aloe in pots on a sunny windowsill.

Aloes have a history of use going back for at least 5,000 years. In Ayurvedic medicine Aloe vera gel is considered to possess estrogenic properties, and this may be one of the reasons the plant was so highly esteemed by Indian, Arab, Egyptian and Mediterranean women. Aloe was known and widely used in Asia, and is found in the folklore of the Japanese, Filipinos and Hawaiians. Its name is derived from the Arabic word *alloeh,* meaning bitter, most likely due to the bitter liquid found in the leaves.

A Sumerian clay tablet found in the city of Nippur, written around 2,200 B.C., documents the first recorded use of Aloe vera as a laxative. A detailed account of Aloe's medicinal value is found in the Egyptian Papyrus Ebers, dated about 1,550 B.C. This document records twelve formulas combining Aloe with other substances for the treatment of both internal and external ills.

Copra's Indigenous Drugs of India, written in 400 B.C. states "The use of Aloes, the common *musabbar,* for external application to inflamed painful parts of the body and for causing purgation are too well known in India to need any special mention."

"Later, Joseph of Arimathea asked Pilate for the body of Jesus. Now Joseph was a disciple of Jesus, but secretly because he feared the Jews. With Pilate's permission, he came and took the body away. He was accompanied by Nicodemus who brought a mixture of myrrh and aloes, about seventy-five pounds. Taking Jesus' body, the two of them wrapped it with the spices, in strips of linen. This was in accordance with Jewish burial customs." John 19:38-40

The master of Roman pharmacology, Dioscorides, 41 A.D.-68 A.D., expanded his herbal knowledge and skill as he traveled throughout the lands with the Roman army. He observed that the whole aloe vera leaf, when pulverized, would stop the bleeding of wounds and attributed to its juices "the power of binding, of inducing sleep." Dioscorides further noted that it "loosens the belly, cleansing the stomach" and was used to treat boils, ease hemorrhoids, heal bruises and dry, itchy skin conditions, was good for the tonsils, gums and mouth irritations, and that it was an effective medicine for the eyes.

By the year 200 A.D. Aloe had become an essential and vital part of Roman medicine.

The plant was brought to the New World by the Spanish in the 1600s. It was planted in gardens and used extensively by the missionaries as well as by the indigenous people as a universal healing agent. Aloe was officially listed as both a purgative and a skin protector by the United States pharmacopoeia in 1820.

During the 20th century countless studies were conducted around the world demonstrating Aloe vera to be therapeutic as well as curative for a wide range of ills. Among them, Aloe has been shown to heal as well as to prevent radiation burns, cut the healing time of fire burns by at least half, and heal ulcers, dermatitis and skin diseases caused by parasites.

Aloe successfully heals cuts, blisters, sores and acne. It greatly improves skin texture and helps eliminate dryness, itching, eczema, psoriasis and other skin diseases, including cancer. Studies have shown that aloe regenerates skin cells, eliminates scarring and promotes regeneration of natural skin color.

It has effectively been used as a treatment for peptic ulcers, lung disorders, chronic leg ulcers, periodontal disease, and seborrhea and hair loss. Aloe is effective against ringworm and other fungal infections, abscess, inflamed cysts and hot spots.

Studies performed in the 1960s and repeated in the 1980s confirmed findings that Aloe is highly effective against *Staphylococcus aureus, Streptococcus viridaus, Candida albicans, Corynebacterium xerosis*, and the five strains of *Streptococcus Mutant,* and that it is nontoxic. Furthermore, Aloe quickly relieves pain, eliminates soreness, irritation and swelling, and is a very effective treatment for herpes and shingles. Researchers concluded that Aloe is a powerful anti-inflammatory and antimicrobial agent and is effective against a broad spectrum of micro-organisms.

Studies conducted at the Chicago Burn Center demonstrated the ability of Aloe vera to heal third degree burns and frost bite up to six times faster than accepted modern medical treatment.

Dr. Heggars, M.D., who directed the study, concluded that these healing effects were due, at least in part, to the steroidal compounds and salicylic acid present in the whole leaf. He found that Aloe eliminated scarring; normal skin color returned, and the hair follicles were completely regenerated, allowing for re-growth of hair in burned areas of the skin and scalp. Aloe was found to be more effective in preventing and controlling infections than Silver Sulfadiazine.

Researchers at the Linus Pauling Institute concluded that drinking Aloe vera juice helps improve protein digestion, promotes balance of digestive bacteria, relieves indigestion and reduces acid stomach. They also found that it helps normalize bowel movements, controls yeast infections, can be a benefit to those dealing with irritable bowel syndrome and colitis, and that it has no toxic effects.

Researchers from Okinawa, Japan, reported in the Japanese Journal of Cancer Research that Aloe contained at least three anti-tumor agents, emodin, mannose and lectin. When Dr. James Duke, the well known herbal educator, was with the United States Department of Agriculture, he approved the use of Aloe mannose as a treatment of soft tissue cancer in animals and of feline leukemia.

A PHARMACY IN A PLANT

Dr. Wendell Winters at the University of Texas Health Science Center in San Antonio reports that Aloe contains at least 140 individual substances. He describes Aloe as "a pharmacy in a plant." Scientists have discovered no less than 70 essential nutrients present, including a wealth of vitamins, minerals, enzymes, protein, phytosterols and amino acids.

Aloe vera juice offers vitamins A (beta-carotene and retinol), B1 (thiamine), B2 (riboflavin), B3 (niacin), B6 (pyridoxine), B12 (cyanocobalamin), choline, vitamin C (ascorbic acid), E (tocopherol) and folic acid; plus the minerals calcium, chlorine, copper, germanium, iron, magnesium, manganese, potassium, silicon, sodium, sulfur and zinc.

The plant also contains the organic acids chrysophanic, salicylic, succinic and uric, and all-important polysaccharides, which are long chain sugar molecules such as acemannen, which act as immune stimulators and anti-inflammatory agents, as well as enzymes such as glutathione peroxidase, and resins.

Phytosterols such as B-sitosterol, a powerful anti-inflammatory and anti-cholestromatic, which helps to lower cholesterol levels, and lupeol, a potent pain reliever and antimicrobial agent are also present.

Among Aloe's ingredients are at least six potent antiseptic agents: lupeol, salicylic acid, urea nitrogen, cinnamonic acid, phenols and sulphur. All of these substances kill or control mold, bacteria, fungus, and viruses which helps explain Aloe's ability to eliminate many internal and external infections.

Aloe also contains at least 23 polypeptides, or immune stimulators, and so is active against a wide range of immune system diseases. These polypeptides, together with the anti-tumor agents Aloe emodin and Aloe lectin, make Aloe an effective ally for the prevention and treatment of cancer.

Acemannan, a constituent of aloe gel shown in laboratory tests to have strong immune-stimulating and potent antiviral activity, is thought to mimic the function of AZT, and is currently being tested as a promising adjunct to AIDS therapy. When 20 ounces of Aloe vera juice was orally administered to 69 AIDS patients per day, symptoms eventually disappeared in 81% of these patients.

Aloe vera is simple to use to treat external conditions, such as burns, wounds and skin afflictions. The clear gel inside the leaf has an immediate soothing effect and places a protective coat over the affected area, speeding the rate of healing and reducing the risk of infection. This action is due in part to the presence of *aloectin B*, another immune stimulating constituent present in the gel. To obtain the gel, cut a leaf in half along its length and apply the inner pulp to the affected area.

The yellow sap that oozes from the base of the leaf when it is cut is called bitter aloes. This bitter sap contains anthraquinones which are a useful digestive stimulant and act as a strong laxative. Anthraquinones also bind to calcium in the urinary tract and significantly reduce urinary calcium crystals. Aloe can be used to prevent stone formation and reduce the size of kidney stones.

Aloe juice, made from both the skin and gel of the plant, may be a useful therapy for those with diabetes type II, as laboratory studies show that it can stimulate insulin release from the pancreas and reduce blood sugar and triglyceride levels in the blood.

Throughout history Aloe juice has been mixed with water, milk, wine, honey and many other substances to make it easier to use and more palatable, with no loss of effectiveness.

Remember that it is the *synergistic* relationship between all parts of the plant that make Aloe vera such an amazing healer. Most authorities agree that there is no single agent responsible for Aloe vera's ability to heal, and therefore using the whole leaf is most effective. In antiquity the whole plant was used, rather than one or another of its parts. The leaves were often ground up and cooked to preserve their medicinal value when traded across long distances. Successful modern studies have used either a combination of the sap and gel, or the whole leaf.

Literally thousands of modern researchers agree that the juice must be pasteurized or even boiled (212 degrees F) to preserve its value. Chemical reference books, including Merck's Index, state that the polysaccharides, glycoproteins, and other significant ingredients have breakdown temperatures well above the boiling point of water. The polysaccharides, for instance, do not begin to break down until exposed to temperatures above 230 degrees Fahrenheit. If you cannot use the whole fresh plant, be sure you choose a well preserved product.

Consumers beware: According to the International Aloe Science Council, most major brands of cosmetic and toiletries touting Aloe vera as an ingredient contain less than two percent Aloe. Most experts agree that a concentration of at least 25% to 40% is necessary for a product to have any benefits.

Cautions: People with an allergy to garlic, onions or other plants of the *Liliaceae* family may have allergic reactions to Aloe. Application of Aloe prior to sun exposure may lead to a rash in sun-exposed areas.

The oral use of Aloe or Aloe latex for laxative effects may cause cramping or diarrhea. Use for over seven days may cause dependency or worsening of constipation after the Aloe is stopped. Ingestion of Aloe for over one year may increase the risk of colorectal cancer. Individuals with severe abdominal pain, appendicitis, ileus (temporary paralysis of the bowel), or a prolonged period without bowel movements should not take Aloe.

Electrolyte imbalances in the blood, including low potassium levels, which can lead to abnormal heart rhythms or muscle weakness, may be caused by the laxative effect of Aloe. People with heart disease, kidney disease, or electrolyte abnormalities should not take aloe internally.

Although topical use of Aloe is entirely safe during pregnancy and breastfeeding, oral use is not recommended.

Household benefits - Aloe plants are believed to offer benefits and protection to the home as well as its inhabitants. They improve air quality, and when grown in pots inside the house, remove toxins from the atmosphere.

And, Aloe vera has a reputation for protecting the home and its inhabitants from the *evil eye*, still very much a concern here in Southern Italia. It is believed that when kept in the kitchen it helps prevent culinary mishaps.

PASSIONFLOWER

Passiflora incarnata

This graceful climbing plant has long been referred to as the *flower of the passion* and has been associated with the Crucifixion of Christ due to the flower's appearance. Its five anthers resemble the five wounds of Christ as he hung on the cross, the filaments represent the crown of thorns, and the calyx resembles the nimbus, or glory, that surrounded his sacred head.

> *The Passion flower long has blow'd*
> *to betoken us signs of the Holy Road*

Passionflowers are an indigenous American herb, with a long history of use, primarily as a nourishing herb for the nervous system. The leaves and flowers offer potent calming and tranquilizing properties. In higher doses they are sedative and pain easing. Passionflower is effective against insomnia and possesses constituents that give it a reliable antidepressant effect. It is soothing to the spirit.

Passion flower is an entirely safe, non-narcotic herb, with mild psychotropic properties, no known toxicity and no known interaction with any pharmaceutical drugs.

It is entirely safe to give to children and is recommended as a remedy to treat attention deficit disorders. It greatly improves concentration and focus and helps the mind to settle down.

Passionflower can be used as a safe, natural and effective substitute for pharmaceutical drugs that affect the brain and/or nervous system and relieve pain.

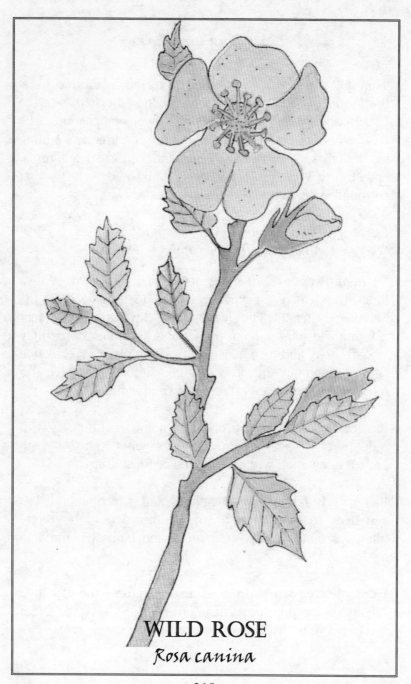

WILD ROSE
Rosa canina

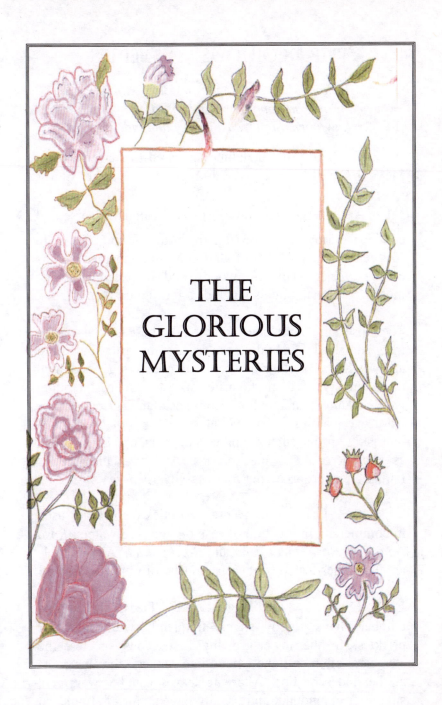

THE GLORIOUS MYSTERIES

THE GLORIOUS MYSTERIES

The Glorious Mysteries center on Mary's Emblem, the Mystical Rose, and on nourishing rose family plants such as hawthorn, apple, strawberry and blackberry.

When Our Lady of Guadalupe appeared to Juan Diego in Mexico, she filled his *tilpa* with fragrant roses as her sign.

ROSACEAE - *The Rose Family* is highly diverse and contains approximately 3350 herb, shrub and tree species in 122 genera, most of them found in north temperate regions of the world. They are woody and herbaceous plants, mostly perennial, but also include a few annuals.

The Rose family includes some of the best known garden trees and shrubs, including the rose, cotoneaster, hawthorn and rowan. It offers a wealth of nourishing, medicinal plants, many of them favorites in the garden, including lady's mantle, marshmallow, hollyhock, and agrimony. The Rosaceae family also includes several of our most nourishing fruits, such as apples and pears, and berries such as strawberries and blackberries. All the plants in this family are appropriate for your Mary Garden.

CHARACTERISTICS: Three varieties of rose are used in commercial production of rose oil and rose waters: *Rosa centifolia*, *Rosa damascena* and *Rosa gallica*. Also notable are the domesticated fruit crops, mostly of Eurasian origin.

LEAVES, STEM AND ROOTS Trees, shrubs and climbers have woody stems, frequently with thorns or prickles. In the lower-growing herbaceous species, the stems are often soft and extend into runners, forming roots at the nodes or tips. Alternate leaves can be evergreen, simple or compound, and usually have a pair of stipules at their base.

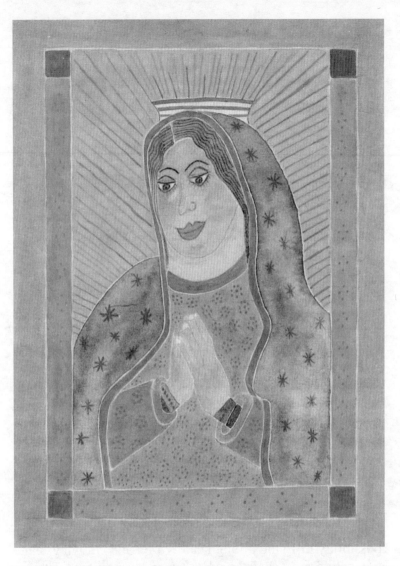

FLOWERS There is a calyx of five sepals, and often another smaller whorl of five sepal-type parts below the calyx (an epicalyx). The individual flowers are often large and showy, but sometimes small and inconspicuous, such as *Alchemilla* and *Filipendula*. They are borne singly, in small clusters or in spikes. There are usually five petals (sometimes four or six), and in cultivated hybrids there may be many more petals. There are many stamens.

SEEDS There are many different types of fruit in the Rosaceae family. The fruit may be a drupe containing one large woody seed (plum, peach, cherry), a collection of drupes, containing several seeds (raspberry, blackberry), a pome, the swollen stem under the flower, containing one or several seeds (apple, hawthorn), a hip (rose), a pseudocarp, a fleshy fruit with achenes on the outside (strawberry), or clusters of achenes with or without feathery tails (geum). The number of seeds varies from a single large stone (plum) to thousands of tiny seeds (*Filipendula*).

FIRST, THE FRUIT-BEARING TREES...

"And God said, Let the earth bring forth grass, the herb yielding seed, and the fruit tree yielding fruit after its kind, whose seed is in itself, upon the earth: and it was so."
Genesis 1

The fruit trees in the Rosaceae family are ancient cultivars that have evolved down through the millennia by natural cross breeding as well as by intentional refinement. Their fruits are common, abundant, nourishing and delicious! They present us with a wide range of nutrients vital for health and well being. Fruits provide us with an excellent foundation for sound and vigorous health; they enhance the possibility of living a long healthy life, and enjoying many grandchildren... People who eat an assortment of fruits have a greatly reduced risk of many chronic diseases.

Regular consumption of fresh, cooked and juiced fruits of the Rosaceae family has been shown to reduce the risk of stroke, cardiovascular disease and type 2 diabetes and to protect against certain cancers, such as mouth and stomach, colon and rectum. In addition, the risks of both bone loss and developing kidney stones are decreased with frequent consumption of fruit.

Most fruits are naturally low in fat, sodium and calories. None have cholesterol and all are important sources of many vitally important nutrients, including potassium, dietary fiber, vitamin C and folic acid.

APPLES *Malus communis* The apple tree originally came from Eastern Europe and southwestern Asia and spread to most temperate regions of the world. Many cultivars have been developed over the centuries, and today there are at least 7,000 varieties of apples.

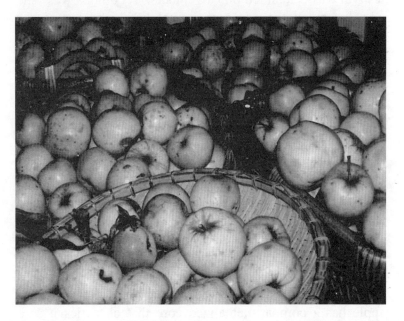

Apple trees were plentiful throughout the ancient world and were among the first of the fruit trees to be cultivated by our early ancestors. The wild apple of the ancients was quite a bit smaller and much tarter than the sweet, juicy apples of today.

Apples have long been associated with the biblical story of Adam and Eve, although there is no mention in the Bible that the tree was actually an apple. Some scholars think the Tree of the Knowledge of Good and Evil was a *sycamore fig*, which represented the Goddess Hathor/Ashorah/Ashtart in all of her resplendent and nourishing generosity. Others surmise it was a *pomegranate*, another fruit tree considered sacred throughout the lands where it grew.

Apples have an ancient association with the Goddess of Love and Abundance and the Goddess of the Harvest. Pomona was the Roman Goddess of fruit trees, especially of the apples. She was called the *Apple Mother* and her festival was celebrated on November 1st. Pomona was "she who bestowed the apple of eternal life," and her sacred grove, located near Ostia, the ancient Roman port, was called the *Pomonal*. All Roman banquets came to an end with the eating of apples and the offering of a prayer for Pomona's blessing.

Traditional American myth tells of the real life person known as Johnny Appleseed. During the early 1800s John Chapman walked barefoot across the plains, covering an area of 100,000 square miles, planting apple seeds. The seeds he planted grew into fruit trees that provided food and a livelihood for generations of early American settlers.

Apples are crisp, white-fleshed fruits with red, yellow or green skin. They range in taste from moderately sweet and refreshing to pleasantly tart depending on the variety. The apple has a compartmentalized core that classifies it as a pome fruit. In the Northern Hemisphere apples are in season from late summer to early winter. During the fall of the year the roadsides and field edges in central Maine are lined with all kinds of wild and colorful apples hanging from the trees. It is a beautiful sight! What does not get picked by humans will become winter food for many animals, especially deer and wild turkeys.

Apples are packed with nourishment! One medium sized apple contains an abundance of vitamins B1 (thiamin), B2 (riboflavin), B3 (niacin), B5 (pantothenic acid), B6 (pyridoxine), B9 (folate) and C, and the minerals calcium, iron, magnesium, phosphorus and potassium, plus much more.

It is wise to remember when reading this type of information, such as the vitamin and mineral content of a fruit or a breakdown of plant constituents in a medicinal herb that we are speaking in reductionist terms, treading on foreign ground. While it is fundamentally important to inform ourselves of what nutrients are available to us and from where, it is equally important to realize that the total value of eating an apple, other fruit or medicinal herb, is greater than the value of the individual vitamins, minerals and phytonutrients it may contain.

It is the *synergy* of these various constituents working together in the wonderfully diverse array that they are presented to us in whole, natural foods and herbs that is the basis of their effectiveness in promoting vibrant health and preventing disease. (The whole is greater than the sum of its parts.)

That said, let's look a bit further into just what apples and these other fruits offer us in terms of specific nourishment.

Some of the health benefits of apples may be related to certain antioxidant phytonutrients they contain, including quercetin, epicatechin and procyanidin. Quercetin is a natural anti-inflammatory chemical, present in many fruits such as apples and herbs such as St. John's wort.

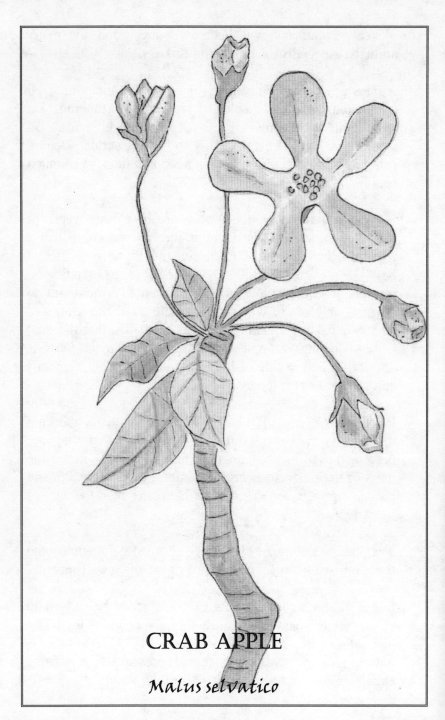

CRAB APPLE

Malus selvatico

It is an anti-allergen and has been used to treat skin and prostate cancers. It has also shown considerable ability to protect the heart. Quercetin is a flavonoid, a substance that gives fruits and vegetables their unique colors. Apple skin and onions are two major food sources of this potent flavonoid.

When quercetin is combined with vitamin C, also found in apples, they become a dynamic antioxidant duo, working together to bolster the body's immune defenses, protecting against cancer and helping prevent free radical damage that leads to heart disease and stroke.

Epicatechin and other catechins reduce plaque build-up in the arteries and may reduce the negative effects of carcinogens.

Procyanidin or proanthocyanidin is strongly anti-inflammatory and beneficial in the prevention of both heart disease and diabetes. These substances help ease the pain and inflammation of rheumatic limbs and joints.

The value of the natural fiber in apples and other fruits and vegetables in the human diet cannot be overstated. Fiber assists with digestive regularity, offers relief from constipation, and helps prevent life-threatening diseases, such as colon and rectal cancer.

Regular consumption of the natural fiber found in fruits also reduces the risk of obesity, diabetes and heart disease. It is important in the treatment and prevention of inflammatory bowel disease, ulcerative colitis, hemorrhoids, Crohn's disease, diverticulitis and other disorders of the digestive and intestinal tract.

Apples are famous for keeping the bowels moving regularly. Both the insoluble fiber in apples and their soluble fiber, pectin, help relieve constipation. The insoluble fiber acts as roughage, and the pectin works as a stool softener by drawing water into the stool and increasing bulk. Because pectin firms up an excessively loose stool, eating an apple is also an effective treatment for diarrhea.

Studies have shown that the phytonutrients found in apples may also protect the brain from Alzheimer's and Parkinson's disease.

Be sure to eat the peel! One medium sized, unpeeled apple provides over 3 grams of fiber, more than 10% of the daily fiber intake recommended. Most of the fiber and many of the most important phytonutrients are found in the apple peel. Studies have shown that eating one apple a day can decrease serum cholesterol by 8-11%.

Pectin is an important health boosting substance found in apples and other fruits in this family, especially pears. Pectin attracts and grabs hold of toxins and heavy metals such as lead and mercury that may be lurking in the bloodstream, and escorts them safely out of the body.

Apples derive almost all of their natural sweetness from fructose, a simple sugar, but one that is broken down slowly, especially when combined with apples' hefty dose of fiber, thus imparting steady energy while helping to keep blood sugar levels stable.

A study published in the *British Journal of Nutrition* found that when women drank ½ to 1 liter of apple, grapefruit or orange juice daily, their urinary pH value and citric acid excretion increased, significantly dropping their risk of forming calcium oxalate stones.

Not all fruit juices are the same. They differ markedly in the variety of phenolic compounds and antioxidant activity. Concord grape juice, *cloudy* apple juice, cranberry juice and grapefruit juice all top the list for health boosting nutrients. Cloudy apple juice was found to contain up to four times the amount of protective polyphenols as clear apple juice.

Studies indicate that long-term fruit juice consumption can provide protection against Alzheimer's disease and suggest that, since each fruit juice contains its own array of protective phenols, drinking a variety of juices may offer the best protection.

However, processing apples into juice greatly lowers their phytonutrient content. Apple juice obtained by pulping and straight pressing was found to have only 10% of the antioxidant activity of fresh apples.

Whole apple extracts, in amounts equal to eating one, three or six apples a day, were shown to prevent breast cancer in test animals in a study published in the *Journal of Agricultural and Food Chemistry*. And apples worked cumulatively: the more apples eaten, the more protection gained.

In another study, published in *Molecular Nutrition and Food Research*, a polyphenol-rich extract of an apple juice blend powerfully inhibited the growth of human colon cancer cells in the laboratory.

The skins of certain cultivars of apples contain high concentrations of antioxidant phenols that not only assist in the prevention of a number of chronic diseases but also appear to provide a hefty dose of UV-B protection. According to a study published in the *Journal of Experimental Botany*, it may be wise to carry along a

Braeburn apple the next time you plan to spend the day in the sun. They accumulate UV-B protective quercitin glycosides in their skin.

One review that analyzed the data from 85 studies found that apples were most consistently associated with a reduced risk of cancer, heart disease, asthma and type 2 diabetes when compared with other fruits and vegetables. Eating apples was also associated with increased lung function and weight loss.

Apples maintain their integrity through long storage times. After 100 days, the amount of phenolic compounds in the skin begins to decrease slightly, but even after 200 days in cold storage, the total amount of these compounds remains close to the level they were when harvested.

Look for firm fruits with rich coloring. Yellow and green apples with a slight blush are best. Your choice of variety depends on your preference for a sweeter or tarter fruit and whether you plan to enjoy your apples raw or cooked.

Red and Golden Delicious are among the sweetest apples and are usually eaten raw. Braeburn and Fuji apples are slightly tart, and Gravenstein, Pippin and Granny Smith apples are the most tart of all. The tart apples retain their texture best during cooking so are preferred for making desserts like apple pie or crisp.

Hildegard of Bingen, one of my favorite herbalists, said that a raw apple is the best food for the healthy, and a cooked apple, the first course of treatment for the ill. To prevent browning when slicing apples for a recipe, simply put the slices in a bowl of cold water to which a spoonful of lemon juice has been added. Sliced apples and cheese are a European favorite.

PEAR *Pyrus communis*

Sweet and juicy, with a soft, buttery texture, pears were once referred to as the "gift of the gods." While the cultivation of pears has been traced back in western Asia for at least three thousand years, most scholars believe that this juicy fruit was enjoyed in its wild form by Stone Age people.

The pear was sacred to Venus and Juno, and statues of Hera were carved in pear wood. Because of its shape, the pear was associated with the female womb and with fecundity. It appears often in images of the Virgin and Child and usually represents sweetness, virtue and all that is good.

Pears were a luxurious item in the court of Louis XIV. The early colonists brought pears to America, and the first pear tree was planted in 1620. Like many other fruit trees, pears were introduced into California and Mexico by Catholic missionaries who planted them in their gardens. Today, much of the world's pear supply comes from China, Italy and the United States.

Pears generally have a large round bottom that tapers towards the top. Depending upon the variety, their paper-thin skins can either be yellow, green, brown, red or a combination of two or more of these colors. Like apples, pears have a core that features several seeds.

Pears are a good source of vitamin C and copper. Both of these can be thought of as antioxidant nutrients that help protect cells in the body from oxygen-related damage due to free radicals.

Vitamin C functions as an antioxidant in all water-soluble areas of the body, and in addition to its antioxidant activity, is critical for good immune function. Vitamin C stimulates white cells to fight infection, directly kills many bacteria and viruses, and regenerates vitamin E (which protects fat-soluble areas of the body) after it has been inactivated by free radicals. Copper also helps protect the body from free radical damage. And pears are an excellent source of that all-important dietary fiber, pectin, as well as vitamin K.

Pears are often recommended as a hypoallergenic fruit as they are less likely to produce an adverse reaction than other fruits. And pear is often suggested as the best fruit to start with when introducing foods to an infant.

While there are literally thousands of varieties of pears, all differing in size, shape, color, taste and storage qualities, the Bosc, Bartlett, Anjou and Comice pears are the most commonly available in the United States.

Since pears are very perishable once they are ripe, the pears you find at the market will generally be unripe and will require a few days of maturing. Look for pears that are firm, but not too hard. They should have a smooth skin that is free of bruises or mold. The color of good quality pears may not be uniform as some feature *russetting,* or brown-speckled patches on the skin; this is an acceptable characteristic and oftentimes reflects a more intense flavor.

Pears should be left at room temperature to ripen. Once their skin yields to gentle pressure, they are ripe and ready to be enjoyed. And again, much of the good stuff is in the skin, so there is no reason to peel it. Once cut, pears will oxidize quickly and turn a brownish color. To prevent this, apply lemon, lime or orange juice to the flesh.

Combine pears with mustard greens, watercress, leeks and walnuts for a delicious salad. Try pears with goat or mozzarella cheese for a delightful dessert.

PLUMS *Prunus domestica*

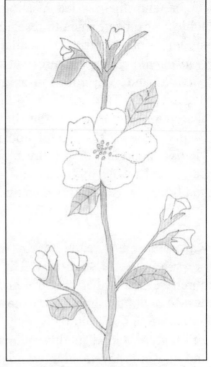

Few fruits come in as many colors as the juicy, sweet tasting plum. Plums belong to the *Prunus* genus and are relatives of the peach, nectarine and almond, all considered *drupes*, because they have a hard stone pit surrounding their seeds. Dried plums are known as prunes.

There are more than 2,000 varieties of plums and about 100 of them are available in the U.S. Plums are classified into six general categories—Japanese, American, Damson, Ornamental, Wild and European/Garden, and each of them vary in size, shape and color. Although usually round, plums can also be oval or heart-shaped.

The European plum originated in the area near the Caspian Sea where it served as a symbol of spring and youth since the earliest times. In Christian iconography the plum usually symbolizes fidelity, but it can also indicate the charity or humility of Christ.

The ancient Italians cultivated more than 300 varieties of plum trees and these eventually made their way across the Atlantic Ocean with the pilgrims, who introduced them into the United States in the 1600's.

Plums and their dried version, prunes, have been the subject of repeated health research for their high content of unique phytonutrients called *neochlorogenic* and *chlorogenic acids*. These substances are classified as *phenols*, and their function as antioxidants has been well documented. The ability of plum and prune to increase absorption of iron in the body is also well known. Plums/prunes' capacity for boosting iron's bioavailability, vitally important for healthy blood and good energy, may be related to the high vitamin C content of this fruit. In addition, plums are a good source of vitamin A (in the form of beta-carotene), vitamin B2, dietary fiber and potassium.

Ripe plums are ready to eat when they yield to gentle pressure and are slightly soft at their tip. While you can purchase plums that are firm and ripen them at home, it's best to avoid those that are excessively hard as they will be immature and it's unlikely they will develop a good taste and texture. Good quality plums will feature a rich color and may still have a slight whitish "bloom," indicating they have not been over handled.

Ripe plums are juicy and delicious eaten as is and can also be cooked in a wide array of recipes. Plums are best cooked by either baking or poaching. They can also be frozen, but to ensure maximum taste, remove their stone pits before placing them in the freezer.

For a yummy plum pizza - broil sliced plums, goat cheese, walnuts and sage on top of a whole wheat pita bread or pizza crust.

Plums are among a small number of foods that contain measurable amounts of oxalates, naturally-occurring substances found in plants. When oxalates become concentrated in body fluids, they can crystallize and cause health problems. Because of this, individuals with existing and untreated kidney or gallbladder problems may be wise to avoid plums. Laboratory studies have shown that oxalates may also interfere with absorption of calcium.

A healthy digestive tract, properly chewing your food and relaxing while you enjoy your meals will ensure you get all the health benefits, including absorption of calcium, from foods that contain oxalic acid.

CHERRIES *Prunus cerasus*

Sometimes called nature's "Super Fruit," the cherry tree was introduced into Italy in the first century B.C. when it was brought back by the Roman army after a military campaign in the southern Black Sea area. Because of their red color, cherries often represent the blood of Christ and sometimes appear on the table in depictions of the Last Supper and in paintings of the Madonna and Child.

Tart cherries, whether enjoyed fresh, dried, frozen or juiced, have some of the highest levels of disease-fighting antioxidants when compared with other fruits. They contain 19 times more beta carotene than blueberries or strawberries, and are crammed with vitamins C and E, potassium, magnesium, iron, fiber and folates.

A recent study conducted by researchers from the University of Michigan Integrative Medicine Program found that cherries in the diet helped reduce risk factors for heart disease and metabolic syndrome, also known as insulin resistant syndrome or pre-diabetes. The study found that consuming cherries regularly helped reduce cholesterol levels, lowered blood sugar levels, and raised the antioxidant capacity of the blood. Called the "silent epidemic" because many of its victims are unaware they have the disease while still in its early stages, metabolic syndrome currently affects nearly one out of four people in the U.S and is increasingly prevalent among young adults.

While there's no clear guideline on how many cherries it takes to reap the benefits, experts suggest 1-2 servings of cherries daily. How much is a serving? At least one big hand full!

Many studies have confirmed that cherries reduce inflammation and pain and offer considerable protection against several serious diseases. Cherries offer benefits for those with autoimmune, neurodegenerative and connective tissue diseases, particularly rheumatoid arthritis and diabetes. These beneficial effects are caused by plant constituents known as anthocyanins.

Anthocyanins are found in both tart and sweet cherries, although levels are higher in the tart varieties. In general, the darker the cherry color, the higher the anthocyanin content.

Scientists at Johns Hopkins University in Baltimore discovered that the anthocyanins in cherries were as effective in reducing painful inflammation as the non-steroidal anti-inflammatory drug, indomethacin. The researchers believe that this effect may stem from the ability of anthocyanins to reduce oxidative stress, which is a major cause of autoimmune disease. Anthocyanin-rich cherries may offer protection against gout, a painful inflammatory condition caused by urate crystals infiltrating joint fluid.

In a related study, researchers demonstrated that tart cherry anthocyanins may also help prevent muscle pain related to intensive exercise. Young men who drank tart cherry juice regularly had decreased symptoms of exercise-induced muscle damage. Tart cherries include the Montmorency and Balaton varieties.

Tart cherries are one of the only natural food sources of the hormone melatonin, which is a potent antioxidant with immunomodulating properties. Cherries are particularly beneficial in reducing the risk of colon cancer. In animal studies of mice prone to colon cancer, the addition of cherries to their diet reduced the number and size of tumors. In other studies cherries diminished the size and growth of breast cancers.

As with pears, plums and apples, the skin of the cherries holds most of the essential antioxidants vital to their health benefits.

BERRIES

Raspberry, strawberry and blackberry, all nourishing and delicious members of the Rosaceae family.

In Old Europe, wild berries were valued as nourishing foods and potent medicines and had a variety of uses. Fresh berry juices were used to create the brilliant and vivid colors used in Medieval frescoes, egg tempera paintings and illuminated manuscripts. During this period only the rich partook of berries' tasty bounty. Today almost everyone has access to fresh, wholesome and nutritious berries in season.

These particular berries are associated with a remarkably long list of health benefits. Besides containing proteins, fats, carbohydrates, and a wealth of vitamins and minerals, they contain several extremely important phytochemicals that help slow down the aging process, boost immunity, and offer protection against a number of chronic diseases. Raspberries, blackberries and strawberries all contain ellagic acid, which research suggests may help to prevent certain types of cancer.

Berries are luscious gifts of nourishment from nature. I love picking the fat, juicy strawberries and plump, succulent blackberries that grow around the edges of our Maine gardens and wildgathering raspberries in the cool shade of the woods during summer. When it comes to berries, fresh off the bush is the absolute best!

These popular berries are naturally sweet and don't require much effort to make into a tasty treat. Just pop them in your mouth as you pick and then bring home the rest, rinse and serve them while they last for a healthy, easy snack or dessert.

Gathering berries from supermarket shelves is fine, just be sure they have been organically grown and look for ripe, colorful, yet firm bodies, with no sign of mold or mushy spots. Getting freshly picked berries in season at farmers' markets, or picking them yourself at a pick-your-own stand, are two great ways to get the freshest berries possible while supporting local agriculture.

Berries can be combined with other healthy foods such as whole grain muffins and bread; just add them as baking ingredients. Jams and jellies preserved with honey instead of the tons of sugar usually called for are delicious when spread on bread or served along with certain meats.

STRAWBERRY *Fragaria virginiana* and *Fragaria chilioensis*.

The strawberry, with its sweet, fragrant flavor, is the most popular berry in the world. Ancient legends say that it sprang spontaneously from the earth during the Golden Age. Strawberries have grown wild for millennia in temperate regions around the world.

There are more than 600 varieties of strawberries and they all differ in flavor, size and texture, though all share the plump, red flesh that has yellow seeds piercing its surface, and the small, regal, green leafy cap and stem that adorn its crown.

King Solomon's crown, and many architectural temple features of the Old World, were inspired by the visual characteristics of this simple little fruit. Strawberries' recorded history goes back at least 2,200 years; the little red berries were highly prized by the Romans and were reported to be growing wild in Italy as far back as 234 B.C.

Strawberries made a big impression in the ancient world. They are mentioned in the writings of Virgil, Ovid, Pliny and later by Shakespeare. Because they were red and juicy, plump and delicious and in the shape of a heart, strawberries were considered sacred to Venus, the Goddess of Love. Later the strawberry was associated with the Blessed Virgin Mary. Strawberry plants appear often in art as a symbol of the Annunciation and the Incarnation of Christ, both of which are celebrated in the spring, when strawberries are in bloom.

In the language of flowers the little white strawberry blossoms represent humility and innocence. In Christian times the red juice of the strawberry was a symbol of the blood, passion and death of Christ, as well as the suffering of Mary.

Medieval stonemasons carved strawberry designs on altars and around the tops of pillars in churches and cathedrals. By the Middle Ages strawberry plants (*F. vesca*) were being transplanted into European gardens for ornamentation, medicine and, of course, for food.

When the first settlers from Europe arrived in Virginia they were overjoyed to find that strawberries, which they referred to as the *wonder of all fruits,* grew wild there.

Ever eaten a double strawberry? Legends say that if you break it in half and share it with a member of the opposite sex, you will fall in love with each other. In France strawberries were long regarded as an aphrodisiac of the highest order. Newlyweds were traditionally served a soup of thinned sour cream, strawberries, borage and powdered sugar to enjoy on their wedding night.

These fruity, heart-shaped valentines are filled with nourishing phytonutrients, including hormone balancing phytosterols. They are a particularly rich source of the phenols, anthocyanin and ellagitannin. These constituents mean that strawberries are a heart-protective fruit, an anti-cancer fruit, and an anti-inflammatory fruit, all rolled into one.

The anthocyanins not only provide strawberries' flush red color, they also serve as potent antioxidants that offer protection to the entire body. The unique *phenols* in this fruit also help to lessen activity of the inflammation-causing enzyme *cyclo-oxygenase*, or COX. Non-steroidal anti-inflammatory drugs alleviate pain by blocking this enzyme, which is implicated in rheumatoid and osteoarthritis, asthma, atherosclerosis and cancer.

The ellagitannin content of strawberries is associated with decreased rates of cancer. In one study, strawberries topped a list of eight foods most linked to lower rates of cancer among a group of over 1,000 elderly people. Those eating the most strawberries were three times less likely to develop cancer compared with those eating few or no strawberries.

Strawberries are an excellent source of vitamin C and manganese. They are also a very good source of dietary fiber and iodine as well as a good source of potassium, folates, riboflavin, vitamin B5, omega-3 fatty acids, vitamin B6, vitamin K, magnesium and copper.

Strawberries are very perishable and should be purchased no more than a few days before being used. Choose berries that are firm, plump, free of mold, have a shiny, deep red color and attached green caps. Since strawberries, once picked, do not ripen further, avoid those that are dull in color or have green or yellow patches, since they are likely to be sour and of inferior quality. Medium-sized strawberries are often more flavorful than those that are excessively large. And the tiny, wild strawberries, as anyone who has ever picked them knows, are the very sweetest of all.

When freezing strawberries for storage, keep them whole, as they will retain much more of their vitamin C content. Canned or otherwise processed berries do not contain anthocyanins; these water-soluble plant pigments are found only in fresh or frozen berries.

Liven up any green salad with freshly sliced strawberries, slivered almonds and a splash of balsamic vinegar. And despite their perishable nature, strawberries hold up very well in fruit salad if properly stored and chilled.

For an easy, elegant dessert, blend fresh or frozen strawberries with a spoonful of honey and some milk or yogurt. Freeze for 20 minutes, then spoon into serving cups and decorate with a sprig of mint.

Cautions: Strawberries are one of the foods most commonly associated with allergic reactions. Other foods associated with allergic reactions include: cow's milk, wheat, soy, shrimp, oranges, eggs, chicken, spinach, tomato, peanuts, pork, corn and beef. The most common symptoms of food allergies include eczema, hives, skin rash, headache, runny nose, itchy eyes, wheezing, gastrointestinal disturbances, depression, hyperactivity and insomnia.

Strawberries are among the 12 foods on which pesticide residues have been most frequently found. Buy and eat only organically grown strawberries.

Strawberries contain measurable amounts of oxalates. Individuals with existing and untreated kidney or gallbladder problems will want to avoid eating large amounts of these fruits. Strawberries also contain goitrogens, naturally-occurring substances that can interfere with the functioning of the thyroid gland. Those with untreated thyroid problems may want to avoid strawberries for this reason.

RASPBERRY

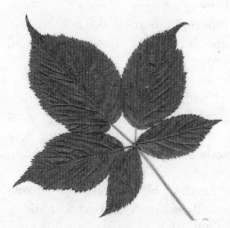

Rubus idaeus is indigenous to Asia Minor and North America. These fruits were gathered from the wild by the people of Troy in the foothills of Mt. Ida around the time of Christ. Records of domestication were found in the 4th century writings of Palladius, a Roman agriculturist, and seeds have been discovered at Roman forts in Britain. The Romans are thought to have spread cultivation of raspberries throughout Europe.

When the settlers arrived in America they found the Native Americans eating indigenous wild raspberries and drying them for preservation. The settlers brought cultivated raspberries with them to the colonies and when George Washington moved to Mount Vernon he began cultivating them in his extensive gardens. One hundred years later more than 40 varieties were known.

Raspberries contain lutein, which is important for healthy vision and protects against macular degeneration. Raspberries are also rich in anti-inflammatory anthocyanins and cancer-fighting phytochemicals, such as ellagic, coumaric and ferulic acids.

BLACKBERRY *Rubus fructicosus*

Blackberries offer special health benefits to women, due to their high concentrations of phytosterols. During studies at the University of Helsinki in Finland, scientists measured eight different berries for their phytoestrogen levels, and concluded that blackberries had the highest levels of these hormone balancing nutrients, followed by strawberries.

Blackberries are considered a valuable astringent because of their high tannin content. Tannins tighten tissue, lesson minor bleeding, and help to alleviate diarrhea and intestinal inflammation. Traditionally, blackberries have been used to shrink hemorrhoids because of their rich supply of tannic acid.

German health authorities recommend blackberries for mild infections, including sore throats and mouth irritations. Scientists have also reported anti-tumor properties associated with the tannins found in some varieties of blackberries. Blackberries are one of the few fruits that contain heart-protective vitamin E. Additional antioxidants in blackberries include vitamin C and ellagic acid; all of these nutrients provide protection against cancer and chronic disease. In fact, blackberries are among the top ten foods containing the highest antioxidant levels.

The brilliant blue/black color of blackberries indicates the presence of the anthocyannin pigment. This substance mitigates more free radicals in the body than any other substance, protects against all kinds of diseases, and acts as a powerful anti-inflammatory agent.

Blackberries are a good source of other phenolic acids, folates and salicylates, the active substance found in aspirin. And, because of their many tiny seeds, blackberries are an excellent source of soluble fiber, such as that all-important pectin.

Blackberries are a superior source of lycopene, another phytochemical that prevents cell damage that can lead to cancer. Blackberries strengthen blood vessels, protect the eyesight and reduce heart disease risk. They offer considerable amounts of potassium, manganese and magnesium.

HAWTHORN *Crataegus spp.*

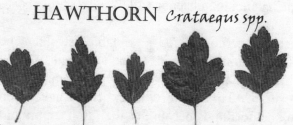

Hawthorn is a spiny tree or shrub indigenous to northern temperate zones of Europe, Asia and North America. The ancient Romans, Greeks, northern Europeans and Native Americans all utilized hawthorn for its heart nourishing properties. Today, it is one of the most commonly used herbs in Europe. Hawthorn is an exceedingly safe and effective long-term heart tonic for maintaining overall cardio-vascular health.

In European countries hawthorn berry extract is considered an effective therapy for mild to moderate congestive heart failure. Hawthorn leaves, flowers and berries are used by herbal practitioners in the UK to treat hypertension in conjunction with prescribed drugs.

Hawthorn contains flavonoids, those wonderful procyanidins and other active compounds. When it comes to the heart and circulatory system, hawthorn is a super star. Regular consumption of hawthorn berries will keep your heart functioning optimally into old age and will especially benefit those with high blood pressure, coronary artery disease, and angina and heart arrhythmia.

European physicians began experimenting with hawthorn for heart disease and other cardiovascular disorders in the early 19th century, and since then its reputation as an effective heart tonic has steadily increased.

Today numerous laboratory tests and clinical trials support this use by demonstrating that hawthorn leaves, flowers and berries contain chemical compounds that increase blood flow to the heart muscle, as well as positively affect other aspects of cardiovascular health.

Hawthorn berries, leaves and flowers improve oxygenation of the blood and brain, which has an immediate beneficial impact on energy levels. Hawthorn's reputation extends to improving blood flow through the heart arteries, increasing the strength of heart contractions and preventing plaque buildup in the arteries.

In addition hawthorn has been found to relax blood vessels so that blood flows more efficiently, help prevent high blood pressure and stabilize collagen. Collagen is the body's most abundant protein and is responsible for maintaining the integrity of the arteries as well as the ligaments, tendons and cartilage. Hawthorn also exhibits anti-inflammatory and anti-oxidant properties.

While there are no acknowledged side effects of hawthorn, it is known to enhance the effects of digitalis, making it more potent. European doctors often prescribe hawthorn to support digitalis and sometimes recommend it as a substitute when digitalis cannot be tolerated or when they want to avoid its side effects. Hawthorn may also increase the effectiveness of beta blocker drugs. If you are being treated for a heart-related condition, be sure to let your physician know if you are considering taking hawthorn, as some of your medications may need to be adjusted.

Hawthorn may best be seen as a heart nourishing herb with preventive properties that can be relied upon to slow down the beginning of cardiovascular damage.

Hawthorn is entirely safe for long-term use and needs to be taken over a period of several months to achieve results. The usual dose is 30-40 drops of tincture three times daily to begin, and then it drops down to twice daily as a maintenance dose after about one month.

The most recent research tells us that our heart is an acutely sensitive organ of perception. Scientists tell us that our heart more closely resembles the brain than a muscle, that it contains millions of neurons, and is in constant communication with the thinking brain. Our heart and brain appear to act in concert, with the heart functioning as the feeling part of our brain.

Learning to open our wild hearts, to connect with the physical earth, cultivating love and compassion for nature, people, plants and animals, touching and being touched, expressing joy and acceptance, all help keep our hearts well toned and functioning optimally.

Heart-healthy foods include fish rich in omega-3 fatty acids, such as sardines, salmon and herring, and flax seed and hemp seed oils. Other foods and beverages that bring a host of benefits to the heart include herbal meads and fermented beverages in moderation; green tea; nuts and seeds rich in essential fatty acids; oatmeal; seaweeds; antioxidant-rich blueberries and other anthocyanidin-rich fruits, such as blackberries, elderberries and grapes; foods rich in carotenes, such as carrots and sweet potatoes; and potassium-rich foods, such as bananas, apples and potatoes.

Some of my favorite herbs for nourishing and toning the heart include motherwort, dandelion, oatstraw, ginkgo, rosemary, angelica, ginseng, ginger, nettles, hawthorn, elderberry, garlic, lemon balm, red clover, willow and rose.

Roses are not only beautiful, they are a sacred and powerful medicine, especially renowned as nourishers of the heart. Both our physical hearts and our emotional hearts respond beautifully to the chemistry and aroma of rose. And our wild hearts open magnificently under the tutelage of these luscious blossoms, as well as their fruit.

There are many reasons that this flower and its fruit were revered by all peoples who knew of and used them. And their especially potent nourishing and protective energies may be one of the main reasons they became associated with Mary, and called the Emblem of Our Lady.

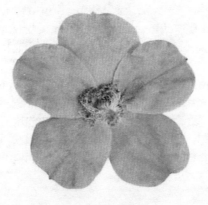

ROSE PETALS & HIPS *Rosa spp.*

Rose petals contain vitamin C, carotene, B complex vitamins and vitamin K. Almost all the minerals listed in the Mendeleyev periodic table are found in rose petals. They offer abundant calcium, so important for strong bones and steady nerves; potassium, important for healthy heart activity; copper, necessary for good functioning of the endocrine glands; and iodine, vital for thyroid gland health.

I've written extensively about the myriad health benefits of roses in two previous books, *Opening Our Wild Hearts to the Healing Herbs* and *Traversing the Wild Terrain of Menopause: Herbal Allies for Midlife Women and Men*.

> *Briefly, roses are a universal symbol of love and an indispensable tonic to the entire body!*

Long considered a symbol of love, roses were sacred to Venus. According to ancient stories, a thorny bush emerged out of the same foamy sea as the Goddess, and when watered by the nectar of the gods, blossomed profusely with beautiful white roses.

Roses were also an attribute of the three Graces, and in Roman times the *Rosalia*, or celebration of the roses, was associated with the cult of the dead. In Christian times the rose became associated with Mary, and still is to this day.

As the Madonna of the Roses, Mary is depicted with the infant Jesus, surrounded by roses, or under an arbor of roses. Roses are also associated with the Immaculate Conception and with the Assumption and Coronation of Mary. Sometimes Jesus holds a red rose, an allusion to his Passion.

ROSES are soothing to the nerves, help relieve emotional upset and act as a mild sedative and antidepressant. I have found roses indispensable for alleviating stress and easing heartache. Rose has a positive influence not only on the nervous system but the brain, the heart and circulatory systems, the bones, the endocrine system, reproductive organs, digestion and immunity.

Roses have an ancient reputation as an aphrodisiac. They enhance fertility in the female and strongly promote it in the male. Men's sperm motility skyrockets when they smell the aroma of rose. Is that why men offer a bouquet of roses when they are in the mood for romance?

Rose petals are antiviral, antibacterial and antiseptic. Bacteria die within five minutes of contact with fresh rose petals. I've used them to heal festering wounds and burns. A tea, honey or syrup made with roses often soothes a mild sore throat. And they are fabulous for the skin.

ROSE OIL   Both rose flower infused oil and rose hip oil are renowned for their benefits for the skin. Rose hip oil in particular has a reputation for eliminating scarring, including acne scars. Rose flower oil helps ease eczema or any red, scaly or itchy skin condition, hydrates the skin and repairs skin cell damage, helps reduce wrinkles and is especially beneficial for dry, mature skin.

ROSE WATER   Roses have a tonic and astringent effect on the capillaries just below the skin surface, so they help diminish the redness caused by enlarged capillaries. Rose water is delightful, easy to make from fresh or dried roses and very soothing to dry, irritated skin. It's a valuable antiseptic for eye infections. And it's a great skin toner, sprayed or splashed on the face after washing. I have used it to help heal a persistent rash on my leg that would not respond to any other treatments.

Our ancient ancestors used rose water to treat upset nerves, and inhaled its steam to treat lung disorders. Rose petals, extracts and syrups of rose were used to treat those with heart pains and kidney diseases.

ROSE HIPS contain the all-important polyphenols anthocyanins, catechin and quercetin. They offer an abundance of health boosting carotenoids, including beta-carotene, lycopene and lutein. Rose hips are bursting with vitamin C, B complex vitamins, vitamin E, chromium, niacin, phosphorus, protein, sodium and zinc. They present us with bioflavonoids, tannins, oils and resins, citric and mallic acids, fructose, saponins, mucilage and pectin as well.

Rosehips have a higher proportion of vitamin C than any other commonly available fruit or vegetable. The content of ascorbic acid in rose-hips is ten times more than in blackcurrant, 50 times more than in lemon and 100 times more than in apples. There is as much vitamin C in a cup of rosehip pulp as in 40 oranges.

I've read that rose hips collected in the north contain more vitamin C than hips collected in the south and that hips exposed to the most sunlight contain the most vitamin C.

To make your rose hip teas and infusions even more effective, add some honey or lemon juice. This becomes a matchless medicine to protect against cold, flu, sore throat, chronic bronchitis and lung distress. It may also ease stomach upset and help heal a duodenal ulcer.

The anti-inflammatory properties of rose hips make them valuable additions to the diets of those with osteoarthritis and rheumatic swellings and pain. Rose hips have been shown to help alleviate pain and stiffness in the knees, hips, and other joints.

Researchers in Denmark divided 94 osteoarthritis patients into two groups. One group received 5g of rose hip powder daily and the other group got a placebo powder for three months. Then they switched powders for another three months. Those taking the rose hip powder reported significant reduction in pain, disability and stiffness. They also reported a marked decrease in the amount of pharmaceutical analgesics they needed to take.

We gather roses at the end of every day while they are blooming and gather the hips in the early fall when they are bright red and plump. I like to thread rose hips into long strands and hang these to dry. Sometimes I dry them, like I do the flower petals, on screens. When completely dry the rose petals and hips can be stored in securely closed brown paper bags.

Roses grow wildly and abundantly all along the coast of Maine, and I make a special trip to the ocean each fall to harvest some of the huge red hips with a salty flair.

While there I usually also look around for some nourishing seaweeds to take home with me, since I love adding them to salads during summer and to soups in the winter. I also appreciate seaweeds for what they do to my skin and hair. And the combination of seaweed and roses in a bath is fantastic!

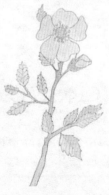

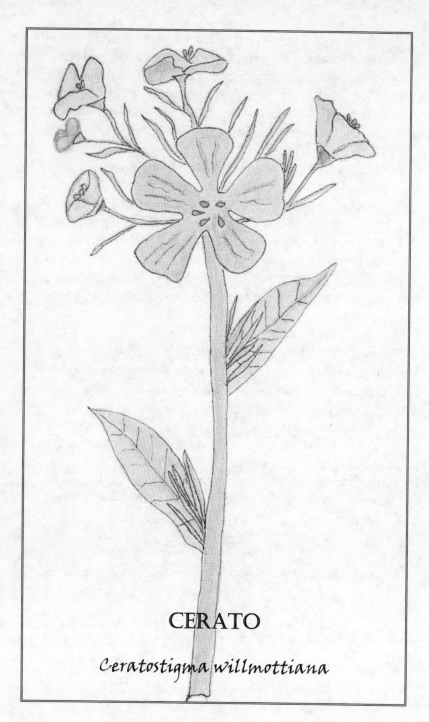

CERATO

Ceratostigma willmottiana

SHE IS THE STAR OF THE SEA

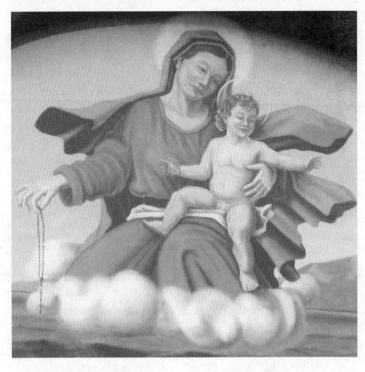

FOOD, MEDICINE AND BEAUTY FROM THE SEA

THALASSOTHERAPY

Hot seaweed baths, wraps and rubs, massages with warm sea water and mud body wraps are some of the essential components of thalassotherapy, a form of health and beauty care widely enjoyed by Mediterranean peoples. Thalassotherapy, derived from the Greek word *thalassa* which means "sea," uses the beneficial aspects of the local marine environment - the climate, sea water, seaweed and algae, mud and sand - for therapeutic purposes. It evolved naturally along with the people who inhabited these coastal areas.

My daughter Rosa and I are dreaming of the day we will take a ferry out to Ischia, an island south of Napoli that is famous for the healing, hot thermal springs that gush up out of the ocean floor. There are also countless *terme*, hot fresh water springs, throughout Southern Italy that are widely used for healing therapies. These thermal waters are said to be rich in essential nutrients that enhance healing and detoxification.

For a super skin nourishing treat, try putting a small handful of dried seaweed into a cotton or muslin bag, or inside a facecloth, wetting it well with hot water under the shower, or in the tub, and then rubbing it all over your body. It's incredibly soothing and skin rejuvenating! Your skin will feel so alive and tingly, clean and healthy afterwards, and it will be glowing.

Or, soak in a seaweed bath. The sea greens help to balance body and skin chemistry. Electrolytic magnetic action of the seaweeds releases excess body fluid from congested cells and dissolves fatty wastes through the skin, replacing them with depleted minerals, particularly potassium and iodine. This is according to Michelle Leigh, author of *Inner Peace, Outer Beauty*, a book about Japanese beauty customs. Leigh adds that the vitamin K in sea vegetables helps regulate adrenal function, thus a regular seaweed bath or rub helps ensure well balanced hormones and a more youthful physical appearance, as well as diminished symptoms of menopausal distress.

And seaweeds are famous for nourishing beautiful, healthy hair, as well as skin. This effect may be due to all those organic colloidal minerals such as silica, calcium, iron and phosphorus, or the emulsifying alginates that cleanse surface toxins and de-acidify, or perhaps it's the abundance of iodine, amino acids and B vitamins…. Seaweeds help remove dirt and excess oil from the hair while imparting a rich supply of the essential nutrients necessary for strong, lustrous, easy to manage hair. You may want to try making a seaweed tea, letting it steep for thirty minutes, then using it as the final rinse over your hair, being sure to massage your scalp as well.

I became very interested in the therapeutic uses of seaweeds while in Italy, and when I returned home to Maine decided to learn more. One bright, mid-July day, four lively and excited apprentices and I packed ourselves into my car and drove down to a little town called Franklin on the coast of Maine. We'd been invited to meet Shep Erhart and have a tour around his Maine Coast Seaweed facility. After being introduced to an array of North Atlantic harvested seaweeds in various stages of drying, processing and storing, Shep led us to one of his favorite places to gather these nourishing local sea vegetables.

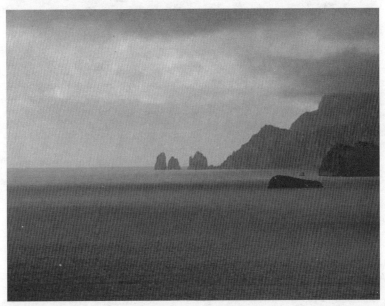

We arrived in a mist, the salty spray of the ocean greeting us, the waves gently breaking on the rocks, the roar like a calming balm. Water birds, or maybe seals, floated on the surface of the water, way out from the shore line.

The ocean was teeming with life, energy and an incredible vitality here in this completely protected, utterly wild and pristine place. Since we purposely timed our visit to coincide with low tide, we found the rocks literally covered with glistening seaweeds of many varieties. And, at the water's edge, where sea meets sand and rock, graceful and supple fronds of seaweeds, holding fast to the bedrock beneath, swayed with the movement of the water, seeming so strong, resilient, tenacious, and absolutely dazzling.

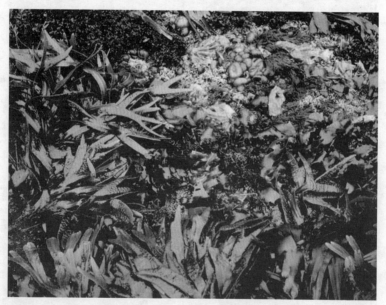

According to Shep, who has been eating, harvesting, working with and enjoying seaweeds for the past thirty years, sea vegetables contain the broadest range of minerals of any food -- the same minerals found in the ocean and in human blood, such as potassium, calcium, magnesium, iron, and iodine. One of the seaweeds we found in abundance on the day we visited was *Luminaria longicruris*, or kelp, a beautiful brown seaweed that grows

4 to 8-foot-long broad golden fronds. Kelp offers exceedingly high amounts of these minerals, and is an unparalleled source of other essential trace nutrients, particularly iodine. "Our cells and those of seaweed are both bathed in a similar ocean of dissolved mineral matter. The ratio of sodium to potassium is nearly the same in blood and saltwater," Shep told us as he gently nudged a bit of seaweed from the rock to give us a closer look.

Kelp has been found to have a normalizing action on the thyroid and parathyroid glands. A healthy, functioning parathyroid gland means you can absorb all those minerals to your best advantage, especially those that play a role in keeping the arterial walls elastic, reducing the risk of hypertension, and normalizing blood pressure. Studies suggest that kelp not only helps to keep both cholesterol and blood pressure down, but also has a positive effect on the balance of healthy flora in the intestinal tract, actively destroys cancer cells, and stimulates T-cell production in our immune systems. These sea vegetables are strongly immune enhancing. Numerous researchers have also discovered kelp's ability to bind with radioactive isotopes in the body, thus allowing them to be safely excreted. Consuming kelp regularly will offer protection to the cells in your body during and after radiation treatments, after any routine x-rays and most especially after any kind of radiation poisoning.

Kelp is a versatile seaweed. It is superb when lightly toasted or fried; it can be pickled in brine or simmered in soups; it's great sautéed; and it's indispensable in bean dishes, as it helps to tenderize beans, shortens the cooking time and aids in digestion.

Sea vegetables have been used for centuries in both Japanese and Chinese medicine, as well as throughout the Mediterranean region, for the treatment of serious diseases, including cancer, and recent scientific studies have verified these uses. Antitumor and antimutagenic activity has been found in the kelps, kumbu and wakame. The polysaccharides extracted from both brown seaweeds and red have been shown to inhibit cell growth, suggesting they may be able to inhibit cancer cell growth as well.

It is well documented that in cultures where seaweeds are consumed regularly, like Japan, and some places along the Mediterranean, the people enjoy very low rates of cancer. Jane Teas, affiliated with Harvard School of Public Health, published a paper three decades ago suggesting seaweeds, specifically kelp, as an important contributing factor to the relatively low breast cancer rates among postmenopausal women in Japan. Teas proposed that kelp plays a major role in both preventing the initiation of breast cancer, as well as inhibiting its promotion.

Another sea vegetable we found anchored to the rocks at the water's edge on this trip was deep, dark red, hand-shaped dulse, *Palmaria palmata*. Dulse is luminescent under water and actually seems to sparkle. It's so pretty! This common red seaweed is delicious, and since we brought a bucket full of dulse home with us, I began finding lots of ways to introduce it into our daily meals. I've added it to all kinds of salads, soups and stir-fries, found that it is great with beans, potatoes and fish and really terrific when eaten as a salty snack all by itself. No need to cook this sea vegetable, it is tasty and ready to eat as soon as it is dried. Shep told us that a quick rinse is all that is necessary to tenderize it a bit before adding it to salads and sandwiches. Dulse's very high protein content, more than 22%, makes it higher in protein than chickpeas, almonds or whole sesame seeds.

If you decide to try to harvest some seaweeds, try to find a clean, protected place to gather from. Do so conscientiously, with the ecology of the area, the health of the entire ecosystem, in mind. Take only a very small portion of what you find. Seaweeds are easy to process. They require a good day or two of drying directly in the sun. Our cedar deck made the perfect drying platform. As soon as they are dry, seaweeds should be packed away in paper or plastic bags or glass jars. But keep them handy so that you can remember to use some every day.

Seaweeds are also fabulous nourishers for both plants and soil. According to Shep's book, *Sea Vegetable Celebration*, seaweed or seaweed-based products "increase seed germination and root development, increase bloom set and size of flowers, relieve stress in plants due to weather, insect attack, drought and frost, increase microorganisms in the soil that fix nitrogen from the air, increase mineral uptake from soil and increase shelf life of fruits and vegetables." Seaweed can be composted, spread directly on the soil, made into a tea and applied to the soil or sprayed on plants, used as mulch or tilled into the soil. No matter how you use it, you will be supplying a broad spectrum of organic micronutrients that will nourish both plants and soil, just as they nourish our bodies, inside and out.

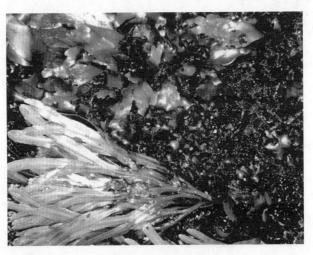

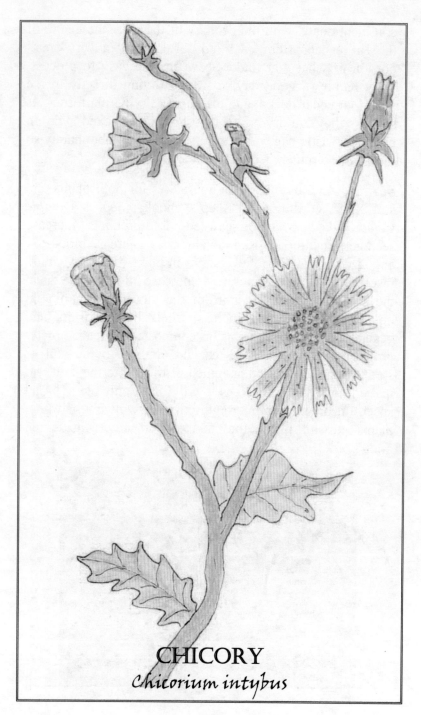

CHICORY
Chicorium intybus

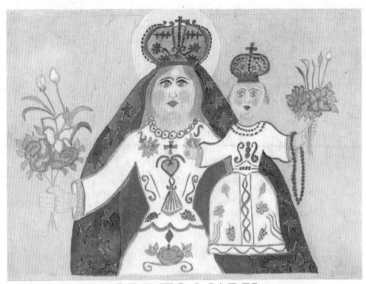

ODE TO MARY

AVE MARIA
My friend
full of grace
When did you come back to me?

I remember kneeling before you often
in St. Peter and Paul Church as a little girl.
You took me up into your arms once to comfort me.
The nuns said you wanted us to pray the rosary
for peace in the world.
So I took it as my responsibility
to say the rosary every night before bed.
All the way up past my teens.
Then I let it go.
For quite a while.

When my children were young I sensed you watching over
and protecting us.
I heard them laughing and playing
and my heart overflowed with love and joy.
I could feel you close by then.

And when my heart heaved and ached and split
into a million pieces?
Your hand on my shoulder,
your words a whisper in my ear.
Words beyond words.
Words of healing, words of beauty, words of grace.

Surely you have been here all along.
But there were years when I rarely thought of you.
Things are different now.
My rosary is never far away,
your prayer is almost always in my heart
and images of you are everywhere
around my home.
Body of Grace
Mother of God
Queen of Heaven
Queen of Peace

More than that, you are alive and vibrant within me,
inspiring my life in a thousand ways.
Day after day.

I've been meditating on you and that son of yours, Jesus.
The fruit of your blessed womb.
You really had your hands full with him, didn't you?
Incarnation of the Word, though he was.
He could be a smart little brat at times we hear.
Staying behind with the teachers in the temple
when he was only twelve.
Causing you such worry!
And so fresh to you at times. Tsk, tsk.
He did have his moments though…
But at Cana, you still ruled Mary.
You let him know who was boss.
And that the time had come, despite his reluctance.
And when you finally did turn him loose
whoa. Now that was something else...

All those healings!
The teachings!
The miracles!
You must have been pleased.
You did so well as a mother.
A consummate, exemplary job!
In fact, everyone is still talking about it.

And then, after all that, standing under the cross.
Fully present as he died in such misery.
Your heart wrenched to see your dearly loved son
in such a state.
Oh, mother!
There are no words for your pain.
There is no remedy for the heartache and sorrow
you have endured.
The greatest painter cannot capture
the anguish and torment in your eyes.

Yet right there and then, you received us.
Took us all in. Silently promised to be ours.
How did your heart get so big?
Was it because you nurtured and gave birth to the
Son of God?
You made him from your own flesh and blood.
Surely that made you more than human.
Blessed among all of us. Yet one of us, still the same.
Much more than a goddess.
You are a woman, you are the Mother of God.
So humble.
Yet so incredibly strong, eager and willing.
That Magnificat! Magnificent!
You were not the least bit afraid to tell it like it was.
Nice job. You are no shrinking violet, that's for sure.

The priests say you are gentle, meek and mild.
They say you are patient, obedient, virtuous and kind.
Yes, but we know that you are so much more than these.

You are the heavens and the stars,
the moon and the earth all rolled into one.
You are the oceans and the streams, rivers and springs.
You are the valley and the mountain and the rainbow.
Lightning and thunder, a maiden's blush.
The winter snow storm and the gentle spring rain.
Wise beyond measure.
In fact, some still say you are Sophia.
We all know you carry Sarah in your veins.

You have so many names, so many faces.
So many attributes and personifications.
You are so illustrious!
And so well traveled...
Our Lady of Guadalupe,
Our Lady of Lourdes,
Our Lady of Fatima,
Our Lady of Mount Carmel,
Our Lady of Czestochowa....Medegorie,
even Brooklyn, New York...
You like to get around!
And make such a lasting impression
wherever and whenever you appear.

And I must say, I absolutely love your outfits!

The star shine and moon glow really suit you.
And that shade of blue, absolutely heavenly!
Though I admit to being partial to your much older
hues of burgundy and red.
I've been meaning to ask, where did you get that beautiful
cloak covered with stars?
Was it from Isis, like some say, or Hera or Diana?

And what about that regal and majestic
jewel-encrusted crown?
Did a former Snake Goddess present that to you when you
arrived on the scene?

For surely all other queens soon faded before your brilliant
and luminous presence.

And that halo?
I'm guessing that was a completely original accessory
designed by and given to you directly by God.
Absolutely stunning! You wear it very well.

You know, Mary, my mother adored you.
So did my grandmothers.
All my aunts and cousins love you
and my daughters do too.
Devotion to you runs in our family.
From way back.
My ancestors have walked on foot
up a narrow mountain trail all night long
to visit you in a cave at its summit
every August 5th sunrise for centuries.
Maybe for thousands of years.
You are in our cells,
You are in our blood
and you are deeply embedded in my heart.

I pray my children and grandchildren know you live in their
hearts as well.
And not just my children,
but all children on earth.

Mary, thank you for helping bring peace to our world.
Viva Maria!
Virgin Mother of God!
Compassionate Queen
Thank you for coming back to me.

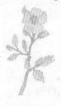

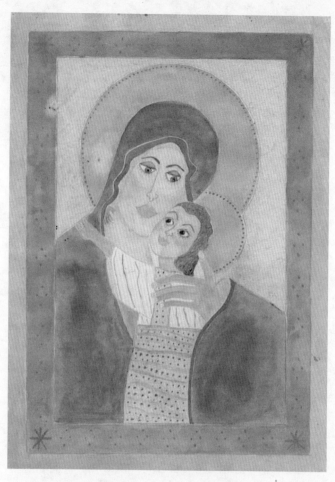

LITANY OF LORETO

Lord, have mercy on us.
Christ have mercy on us.
Lord, have mercy on us.
Christ, hear us.
Christ graciously hear us.
God, the Father of heaven, have mercy on us.
God the Son, Redeemer of the world, have mercy on us.
God the Holy Ghost, have mercy on us.
Holy Trinity, one God, have mercy on us.
Holy Mary, pray for us.
Holy Mother of God, pray for us.
Holy Virgin of virgins, pray for us.
Mother of Christ, pray for us.

Mother of divine grace, pray for us.
Mother most pure, pray for us.
Mother most chaste, pray for us.
Mother inviolate, pray for us.
Mother undefiled, pray for us.
Mother most amiable, pray for us.
Mother most admirable, pray for us.
Mother of good counsel, pray for us.
Mother of our Creator, pray for us.
Mother of our Savior, pray for us.
Virgin most prudent, pray for us.
Virgin most venerable, pray for us.
Virgin most renowned, pray for us.
Virgin most powerful, pray for us.
Virgin most merciful, pray for us.
Virgin most faithful, pray for us.
Mirror of justice, pray for us.
Seat of wisdom, pray for us.
Cause of our joy, pray for us.
Spiritual vessel, pray for us.
Vessel of honor, pray for us.
Singular vessel of devotion, pray for us.
Mystical rose, pray for us.
Tower of David, pray for us.
Tower of ivory, pray for us.
House of gold, pray for us.
Ark of the covenant, pray for us.
Gate of heaven, pray for us.
Morning star, pray for us.
Health of the sick, pray for us.
Refuge of sinners, pray for us.
Comforter of the afflicted, pray for us.
Help of Christians, pray for us.
Queen of Angels, pray for us.
Queen of Patriarchs, pray for us.
Queen of Prophets, pray for us.
Queen of Apostles, pray for us
Queen of Martyrs, pray for us.
Queen of Confessors, pray for us.
Queen of Virgins, pray for us.
Queen of all Saints, pray for us.
Queen conceived without original sin, pray for us.
Queen assumed into heaven, pray for us.
Queen of the most holy Rosary, pray for us.
Queen of Peace, pray for us.

Lamb of God, who takes away the sins of the world,
spare us, O Lord.
Lamb of God, who takes away the sins of the world,
graciously hear us O Lord
Lamb of God, who takes away the sins of the world,
have mercy on us.

Pray for us, O holy Mother of God.
That we may be made worthy of the promises of Christ.

LET US PRAY

Grant, we beseech Thee, O Lord God, unto us Thy servants, that we may rejoice in continual health of mind and body; and, by the glorious intercession of Blessed Mary ever Virgin, may be delivered from present sadness, and enter into the joy of Thine eternal gladness. Through Christ our Lord. Amen.

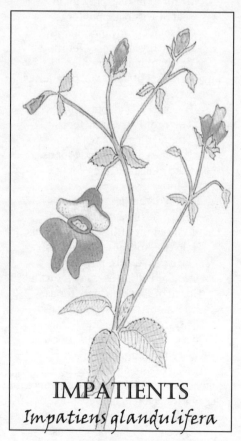

IMPATIENTS
Impatiens glandulifera

Epilogue

Hidden within the heart of the Universe
A gem
It is you and I and all of life
Thriving
Pulsing
Being part of our biosphere
Nothing more
Each of us the very center
of the Universe
Nothing less
It's been proven
By astrophysics!

THE HEARTH FIRE, HESTIA'S GIFT

The hearth fire plays a central role in the homes, as well as the hearts, of the people here in our little village. Though the hearth styles vary, from the most humble and basic, to the truly ornate, they all have the same essential function, which is to provide heat and comfort for the home. In the early morning hours I love watching curls of smoke rise from the chimneys above all the orange tile roof tops. Every chimney fixture is also quite distinctive, each one an artistic representation of the people who reside in the home. It seems that everything the people of my beloved Italian village do, they do with an artful flair.

Our fireplace, like most of the others, is located in the middle of the kitchen, placed not only for heating but for cooking as well. All of the charming stone houses that line the narrow cobblestone passageways here in the historic part of the village where we have our home were built during the Middle Ages, long before gas stoves were invented. So the fireplace is also where our people have always done, and often still do, their cooking. What's more, it is where you will find nearly everyone sitting around during the winter months on little wooden chairs, enjoying each other's company and the cozy warmth of the fire. My daughters and I have spent many happy hours doing nothing more than sitting by our hearth fire in the evenings. And I love the daily meditation of preparing the fire, gathering together my wood for the morning ignition, placing the sticks just so, and as needed, to keep the fire blazing, and the warmth radiating, watching the flames climb as they consume the precious fuel.

Yes, wood is considered precious among the people of our village, as in nearly all places around the world. Acquiring and bringing in wood is hard work, and one more of the soul-nourishing customs of these people I have come to love so dearly. My experience recently brought home to me all the more clearly just how precious wood really is. And how deeply representative the connection is between heart and hearth.

Since our supply of firewood was rapidly dwindling, we made arrangements to have a new load delivered. Our modest house is tucked away in a sweet little courtyard, inaccessible by truck or tractor, or even a car for that matter. The nearest you can get with any driving machine is up the cobblestone steps and around a little hill, so getting wood here is no easy matter. I was expecting the firewood to arrive in the morning and planned that when my daughter Belle returned from school in the afternoon the two of us would work at carrying the wood over to our house together. I was totally unprepared for the events that followed.

A loud rapping at the door first alerted me to the day's unfolding. It was Antonia, our neighbor just outside the courtyard and directly across from the ancient stone archway that leads to our house. Antonia is a striking 95-year-old woman; very thin and tiny; a widow, so dressed entirely in black; vibrant, lively, and with an absolutely beatific smile. In the usual rapid-fire speech pattern of the San Giacomese dialect, she excitedly told me, while gesturing vividly with her arms and hands, that my load of wood had arrived. Grabbing my arm and pulling me out the door, and up the cobblestone pathway, she showed me the pile, a big jumble of 2-foot-long sticks of wood of various thicknesses, which had been unloaded just minutes before and was completely blocking the pathway.

Together, as she muttered her annoyance at the disarray, we threw all the stray sticks on top of the rest of the pile to clear a narrow passageway for walking. Another neighbor up above, Antonia's daughter-in-law, Francesca, had also gotten a full load of wood delivered this morning, and equipped with a sturdy looking pair of gloves on her hands, was busy lugging and stacking it in her wood shed. Once the pile was cleaned up a bit, I asked them both if it would be alright to leave it as it was until my daughter returned from school to help me bring it in. "Si, si" they said, cheerfully nodding and smiling.

Antonia was now chatting away to me, gently poking me on my chest, as she usually does, joking and lavishing her affection on me with every word and gesture. Her daughter-in-law called over to her, "no capito, no capito" (she doesn't understand you) and Antonia turned toward her, a flicker of impatience in her voice, and shouted words I didn't know, but, again, were very clear. "Of course she understands me, she understands everything I say to her, *signora Americana* is my friend." She then turned back to me grinning, proudly grabbed hold of my arm and walked me down to her door, where we parted after a big hug.

I am so fortunate! I have been blessed with the best neighbors in the world here! (And not just here, but home in Maine also.) They are loving, fun, generous and unbelievably kind. You see, at this time it was difficult for me to walk independently. My right ankle, sprained and twisted, had to be supported by a brace. Thankfully, I was still able to get around with the help of an olive wood cane. This had not gone unnoticed by my neighbors.

When my daughter Belle arrived home from school, and I opened the door for her, I saw that a wheelbarrow had been parked right outside my door by Carmella, with whom I share the courtyard. My next door neighbor Carmella is no stranger to hard work. In fact, she seems to thrive on it. Carmella is 73 years old, and as is the case with most of the elder people here, is incredibly strong and vigorous. Able to do substantial labor for hours on end, she works in her garden all day long, hoeing, weeding and picking, takes care of her rabbits and chickens, scraping out all their pens daily, and generally does more physical work in a day than the average American does in a week. Still, she is always ready to go to the evening rosary and mass at the Sant Giacomo church, every night, without fail.

So as Belle and I left our house to begin the work of bringing in that big pile of wood, so did Carmella. She was ready and waiting to assist. She bent over that pile as though it were her own, and got right to the work of gathering up armloads and piling them in such as way that my daughter could load them onto the wheelbarrow and push the load down the steps and into the courtyard to be dumped in front of our house. Carmella would not let me carry any wood! Though I resisted, and defiantly grabbed a few armloads, shouting back at her to stop doing our work, she would hear none of it. She stubbornly persisted, piling up the wood for my daughter, and shouting orders at her all the while, how much to load and just how to push so that her shoulders wouldn't hurt later, and so on. My only acceptable position, it became quickly apparent, was in front of the house. As my daughter dumped each load, my job was to gather it up and stack it, neatly. The small pieces on the right, larger ones on the left. Carmella even came over to inspect my progress, to make sure that I was doing it right!

Antonia came out of her door, performing her part by encouraging my daughter as she passed, but not until after she had called her grandson to assist. Within a few minutes Domenico, a strapping 21-year-old, took over the wheelbarrow, and Belle and Carmella worked together to stack up the piles and load it up for him. Domenico now dumped the load in front of the house, and I continued stacking it. Another little while passed and things changed again. Now Carmella was in front of the house helping me stack the wood, and Francesca had joined the party. She was lugging over, one by one, the very largest pieces of wood, even though she had already spent a large part of her day stacking her own load of wood! She designed a strategy for constructing the end of the pile, taking small pieces of wood and laying them crossways, so that the larger pieces lay evenly and would not fall down. My daughter came over at one point and whined, "Ma, every senior citizen in the area is up there now, all telling us the best way to carry this wood in!" All I could do was laugh, and keep stacking, before Carmella took over my job completely.

It wasn't long before the entire pile of wood was ever so tidily stacked in front of our house, a mound of fuel that most of our neighborhood had taken some part in. With lots of smiles, approving nods and looks of satisfaction, the members of our spontaneous work party finally dispersed and went their separate ways. All except Carmella. She held up a finger, saying *"un altimo"* (one minute), disappeared into her cellar and shortly returned hauling out a huge, thick piece of plastic to cover the wood. She proceeded to tell us that she found this plastic in

Buonabitacola, a village quite some distance away, and knew as soon as she saw it that it would serve her well. She tied it up tightly, carried it down that mountainside on her head, and then loaded it on a bus to get it home. I shook my head, beaming at her, amazed by yet another feat of this amazing woman, and the three of us proceeded to get the plastic tucked neatly over the stack of firewood, most of the large sheet still carefully folded at one end.

Satisfied that the job was now completely finished, we stood back and admired our work. It was done. There was one bundle of 4-foot-long, thin sticks, nice and dry, tightly tied together with string, and meant to be used as kindling wood, which my nephew, Angelo, had carried over to me on his shoulders a few days earlier, left stacked outside the plastic on the other side of our door.

That evening I sent my tired daughter down to the *Panificio* (bread store) for some loaves of freshly baked bread to give to my neighbors, as a thank you for their help. *"Niente, niente"* (it was nothing) they kept saying, but looks of appreciation covered their faces. When my daughter and I finally sat resting by our evening hearth fire, we were feeling so good. So happy. Very much at home. But it wasn't over yet.

The next morning, shortly after Belle left for school at about 7:30, I heard what sounded like a loud banging outside. Boom, boom, boom. I couldn't tell from under the warm covers in my cozy bed, just where the sound was coming from, but figured some neighbor was pounding something, somewhere nearby. Half an hour or so later I got up, and as usual went outside to gather up some of those thin sticks to get my morning fire started. I was completely stunned by what I saw. Someone had chopped every stick in that entire kindling bundle in half and stacked them all next to the big pile of wood under the sheet of plastic! And the string that had held them together was placed meticulously to the side of the stack! Who could have done such a thing? Carmella's door opened just then and I heard strains of the *Radio Maria* broadcast she listened to every morning emanating from her house. I had an inkling.

Out she came into the courtyard with a sheepish smile on her face. I said "Carmella, *chi fare questo?*" (Who did this?) and she smiled a little broader and I knew for sure that it was her. She pointed to the dark clouds over head. "*Piove,*" she said, "*piove.*" It was going to rain. She didn't want those long dry sticks to get wet, and they were too long to put in my tiny shed or under the plastic…So she chopped them up for me! At 7:30 in the morning while I was still in my bed! I raised my voice, I'm sorry to say, I actually yelled at her. "What did you do that for? It wasn't necessary." She ignored my yelling, continued smiling and repeated the well worn phrase, "*niente, niente,*" it was nothing.

I stood there speechless, a wild mix of emotions rolling over me. I felt baffled, humbled, amazed and astounded that she would do such a thing. Finally, I surrendered to her tender hearted benevolence and said, "You're 73 years old, what makes you so strong, so good, so kind?" She pointed to her heart and then up to heaven. Her words were unintelligible, but her meaning was very clear. "I get my love and strength from the heart of God." And then I started to cry. Overwhelmed by her thoughtfulness and pure goodness, tears just poured from my eyes, down my face. I couldn't stop them. It was all too much. Too much kindness, too much caring, too much love.

So you see, the hearth fire here in this little medieval village represents in many ways the heart of the people who live here. And the wood we burn in these hearths *is* very precious. It is made all the more precious and dear by the kindness of neighbors who come out of their doors to help bring it in, by the love presented and the care taken by people we didn't even know just a few years ago. Sitting by our hearth fire that night, listening to the thunder rumbling overhead and the rain pouring down on the roof top, we were warmed and comforted, not only by the heat of the burning fire, but also by the awareness of that love offered so abundantly.

I sometimes feel I have a very long way to go to be truly worthy of such neighbors. But in the end, it may be as Elizabeth Gilbert said in *Eat, Pray, Love:* "*Maybe we must all give up trying to pay back the people in this world who sustain our lives. In the end, maybe it's wiser to surrender before the miraculous scope of human generosity and to just keep saying thank you, forever and sincerely, for as long as we have voices.*"

SINCERE ACKNOWLEDGEMENT & THANKS

My family is my treasure and an immense source of nourishment and joy for me. I offer my earnest and heartfelt thanks to each of you for the unique part you play in sustaining and giving meaning to my life; Rosa, Johnny, Kasia and Alex, Grace, Belle and Jack.

Special thanks to Rosa who cared for me while I painted and wrote over several winters in Italy, to Belle who meticulously verified Latin names of all the plants for accuracy and to Grace for the photo of the village that opens these pages.

My Central Maine community is home to many old and dear friends and extended family whose love and support enrich my life. Bouquets full of gratefulness to all of you, especially Fang and Abby, Carol and Michael, Bianca,

Gerda, Paula, the Harlow family, Fay and Joe, Jim's Variety, the folks at FEDCO, all my West Athenian neighbors and my Common Ground Fair community. Special welcome & appreciation to Adamo, Alex and Ben.

Alla mia famiglia, i vicini e gli amici di Monte San Giacomo, specialmente Pietro, Rino e Anna, Angelo, Iolanda, Carmela, Rosina, Maria, Francesca, Antonia, Angela e Pietro, Antonietta, Antonio e Pasquale al Palazzo Marone. Molto grazie. Grazie anche al parroco della parrocchia di "San Giacomo Ap." di Monte San Giacomo, le suore della Scuola dell'Infanzia, ed a tutte le donne che vanno dire il rosario in sere per la loro ispirazione. Mille grazie a Claudia Cardillo di MediaSteno.

A book is in many ways like a garden - it requires the tending of many hands. Sincere thanks and appreciation to Jean English and Tamothy Louten for the significant time, thought and attention they both gave to this work. Gratitude is also offered to Sue Stultz and Ruby Webber who read the early manuscript and offered feedback, and to Brynne Butler for corroborating flower names and researching grain and vegetable binomials. Grateful appreciation is also presented here to Dr. James Duke, and Deb Soule for offering their words of encouragement and support. And a warm, heart felt thank you to Michael J. Caduto for writing the preface.

Finally, respectful acknowledgement is extended to the following authors whose work and wise words are quoted herein: Alvah Simon, Maria Gimbutas, Merlin Stone, Charlene Spretnek, Erla Zwingle Bruce Lipton, Stephen Harrod Buhner, Leonard Shlain, Sue Monk Kidd, Stu Silverstein, Shep Erhart, M. Basil Pennington, Sandor Ellix Katz, Marvin Meyer, Paul Pitchford, Elizabeth Gilbert, Jean Shinoda Bolen, Carol Schaefer and the Grandmothers, Agnes, Tsering Dolma Gyaltong and Flordemayo.

SELECT BIBLIOGRAPHY

THROUGH THE WILD HEART OF MARY
Teachings of the 20 Mysteries of the Rosary and the Herbs and Foods Associated with Them

The Jesus Papers. Michael Baigent, HarperCollins, N.Y., 2006

Calling the Circle, Christina Baldwin, Bantam Books, N.Y., 1994

Catholic Traditions in the Garden, Ann Ball, Our Sunday Visitor Publishing Division, Huntington, Indiana, 1998

Compendium of the Catechism of the Catholic Church, Pope Benedict, United States Conference of Catholic Bishops, Washington, D.C., 2006

The Millionth Circle, Jean Shinoda Bolen, M.D., Conari Press, Berkeley, Ca., 1999

Urgent Message from Mother, Jean Shinoda Bolen, Conari Press, York Beach, Maine, 2005

Goddesses in Older Women, Jean Shinoda Bolen, Harper Collins Publishers, New York, 2001

Secret Teachings of Plants, Stephen Harrod Buhner, Bear & Company, Rochester, Vt., 2004

The Lost Language of Plants, Stephen Buhner, Chelsea Green Publishing, Vt., 2002

Everyday Herbs in Spiritual Life, Michael J. Caduto, Sky Light Publishing, Vt., 2007

Sacred Circles, Robin Deen Carnes and Sally Craig, Harper, San Francisco, 1998

Mary Magdalene, Bruce Chilton, Doubleday, 2005

Aloe Myth Magic Medicine; Aloe Vera Across Time Bill R. Cook, Odus M. Hennessee, Universal Graphics, 1989

The Wild Mother, Elizabeth Cunningham, Station Hill Press, N.Y., 1993

The Secret of the Rosary, St. Louis De Montfort, Montfort Publications, N.Y., 1954

Praying the Rosary, Michael Dubruiel and Amy Welborn, Our Sunday Visitor Publishing Division, Indiana, 2003

Opening Our Wild Hearts to the Healing Herbs, Gail Faith Edwards, Ash Tree Publishing, N.Y., 2000

Traversing the Wild Terrain of Menopause, Gail Faith Edwards, Bertha Canterbury Press, Maine, 2003

Personal unpublished notes, Gail Faith Edwards, 1990 - 2008

Sea Vegetable Celebration, Recipes Using Ocean Vegetables, Shep Erhart and Leslie Cerier, 2000

Campania Art and Archeology, Patrizia Fabbri, Casa Editrice Bonechi, Florence, Italy, 2002

Nourishing Traditions, Sally Fallon, New Trends Publishing, Washington, D.C., 2001

The Liturgy of Flowers in a Mary Garden, Andrea Oliva Florendo, Rosetti Della Vergine Books, New York. 2004

The Golden Bough, Sir James George Frazer, Collier Books, N.Y., 1922

Flower Lore, Hilderic Friend, Para Research, Inc., Rockport, Ma., 1981

Eat, Pray, Love, Elizabeth Gilbert, Penguin Group, New York. 2006

Language of the Goddess, Marija Gimbutus, Thames & Hudson, N.Y., 2001

Goddesses and Gods of Old Europe; Myths and Cult Images, Marija Gimbutus, University of California Press, Berkeley, Ca.

The Living Goddess, Marija Gimbutas, edited and supplemented by Miriam Robbins Dexter, University of California Press, Berkeley, 2001

The White Goddess, Robert Graves, The Noonday Press, N.Y., 1948

Garlic, Garlic, Garlic, Linda and Fred Griffith, Houghton Mifflin Co., Boston/N.Y., 1998

Israeli Site Reveals Ancient Use of Grains, Flour Making Predated Crop Growing, Guy Gugliotta, Washington Post, 5/5/2004; Pg A03

Last Hours of the Iceman, Stephen S. Hall, National Geographic Magazine, July, 2007

Mary; A Flesh and Blood Biography of the Virgin Mother, Lesley Hazelton, Bloomsbury Publishers, N.Y. 2004

Plant Spirit Shamanism, Ross Heaven and Howard G. Charing, Destiny Books, Rochester, Vt., 2006

Cilento, Giampiero Indelli, Fulco Pratesi, L'Airone Di Giorgio Mondadori, Milano, Italy,1999

History of Art, H.W. Janson, Harry N. Abrams, Inc., Publishers, New York, 1966

The Secret Life of Bees, Sue Monk Kidd, Viking Penguin, New York, 2002

The Gospel of Mary Magdala, Karen L. King, Polebridge Press, 2003

Witchcraft in Europe, 1100-1700: A Documentary History, Alan Charles Kors and Edwards Peters, University of Pennsylvania Press,1972

Healing Plants of the Bible History Lore & Meditations, Vincenzina Krymow, St. Anthony Messenger Press, 2002

Mary's Flowers, Vincenzina Krymow, St. Anthony Messenger Press, Cincinnati, Ohio, 2002

Inner Peace, Outer Beauty, Michelle Leigh, Citadel Press, 1995

The Biology of Belief, Bruce H. Lipton, Mountain of Love Books, Santa Rosa. 2005

The Rosary with Fra Angelico and Giotto, Domenico Marcucci, Fathers and Brothers of the Society of St. Paul, N.Y. 2000

Mary, Mother of All Nations, Megan McKenna, William Hart McNichols, Orbis Books, N.Y., 2000

The Gospels of Mary, Marvin Meyer, Ester A. De Boer, Harper Collins, San Francisco, 2004

Contemplating with Mary the Face of Christ, The Rosary of Pompeii, Edited by Pasquale Mocerino, Industria Graffica Sannita, Italia, 2004

The Origins of Man, E.J. Mundell, Health Day Reporter

The Mystical Language of Icons, Solrunn Nes, William B. Eerdman's Publishing Company, Michigan, 2004

Shakti Woman Feeling Our Fire Healing Our World, Vickie Noble, Harper, San Francisco, 1991

A Mystic Garden, Gunilla Norris, Bluebridge, 2006

Mary Through the Centuries, Jaroslav Pelikan. Yale University Press, New Haven, 1996

Praying By Hand, M. Basil Pennington, Harper Collins Publishing, San Francisco, 1991

Healing With Whole Foods, Paul Pitchford, North Atlantic Books, 1993

Witchcraft in England, 1558-1618, Barbara Rosen, University of Massachusetts Press, 1991

Nature and Its Symbols, Translated by Stephen Sartarelli, The J. Paul Getty Museum, Los Angeles, 2004

Grandmothers Counsel the World, Carol Schaefer, Trumpeter, Boston, 2006

The Alphabet Versus the Goddess, The Conflict Between Word and Image, Leonard Shlain, Penguin, 1999

Bread on Earth, Stu Silverstein, Robin Hood Books, Maine, 1994

North to the Night, Alvah Simon, Broadway Books, New York, 1998

Missing Mary, Charlene Spretnak, Palgrave Macmillan, 2004

The Resurgence of the Real, Body, Nature and Place in a Hypermodern World, Charlene Spretnak, Routledge, 1999

Lost Goddesses of Early Greece, Charlene Spretnak, Beacon Press, Boston, 1978

The Goddess in the Gospels, Margaret Starbird, Bear & Company, N. M., 1998

Magdalene's Lost Legacy, Margaret Starbird, Bear & Company, Vt., 2003

When God Was a Woman, Merlin Stone, Harcourt Brace Jovanovich, Publishers, New York, 1976

Icons and Saints of the Eastern Orthodox Church, Alfredo Tradigo, translated by Stephen Sartarelli, J. Paul Getty Museum, Los Angeles, 2004

The Romantic Story of Scent, John Trueman, Doubleday, N.Y., 1975

Alone of All Her Sex, Marina Warner, Vintage Books, New York, 1983

Circle of Mysteries, Christin Lore Weber, Yes International Publishers, 1997

Italy Before the Romans, Erla Zwingle, National Geographic Magazine, January 2005

Pompeii, A Day in the Past, Edizioni Spano, Isernia, Italy, 2005

~

Blessed Maine Herb Farm

MOFGA/USDA Certified Organic Medicinal Herb Products

of impeccable quality

www.blessedmaineherbs.com